The Methuselah Effect

How the Trend Toward Longevity Is Accelerating…

… And Soon Will Turn Your World Upside Down

Patrick Cox

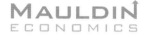

MAULDIN
ECONOMICS

The Methuselah Effect
How the Trend Toward Longevity Is Accelerating...
... And Soon Will Turn Your World Upside Down

Patrick Cox

ISBN: 978-1-365-36730-4

Published by:
Mauldin Economics, LLC
PO Box 192495
Dallas, TX 75219

www.mauldineconomics.com

Dedication

I'm so old, I remember things that aren't on the internet. One of them, I believe, is Samuelson's razor, named for the economist Robert Samuelson. His razor, if my neurons still retain reliability so many years later, was something approximating, "If my wife doesn't understand something I've written, it's not true."

In that spirit, I dedicate this book to my wife Sheryl. A biologist and intelligent skeptic, as opposed to the barren skeptics criticized by Louis Pasteur, she is my plumb line.

Contents

Foreword

I met Patrick Cox a decade ago after seeing a copy of his newsletter on biotechnology and how it is remaking human society and spawning new investment opportunities. I was already interested in technology and transformation, so I was an easy catch for him. I began reading everything he wrote.

Of course, I had questions. I'm not quite certain how it happened, but we began a conversation that quickly grew into a friendship. For the past 10 years, we've been talking every week, and what I've learned from this extraordinary man has given me a new and healthier life.

Patrick's background is Zelig eclectic. He grew up on an Indian reservation where he absorbed a trove of historical lore. He was present at the birth of Netscape and other Silicon Valley pioneers. He plotted strategy with the inner circle of a presidential campaign, wrote for big-time publications, such as *USA Today* and *The Wall Street Journal*, and was a pal of Robert Heinlein. The number and the range of great minds he has collaborated with over the years is astounding—including Milton Friedman, Isaac Asimov, and others I wish I'd had the opportunity to sit down with.

But that's the past. His passion is the future, and his obsession is biotechnology and its growing power to slow human aging. He and I share the view that aging is a malfunction, like a disease, that can be fixed.

Remember, we began talking about this some 10 years ago, and during that time, science has made enormous strides in understanding the biochemical drivers of aging. Out of that understanding have come regimens for slowing the aging process and the beginnings of technology for reversing it. While Patrick and I are hopeful that the final triumph will come during our lifetimes, we are confident that it will happen in the lifetimes of our children.

We don't know his name, but the first person who will reach age 150 is alive today. Patrick and I would like to be around to whoop it up at his big ONE FIVE O party, and because we follow what's happening in biotechnology so closely and know the scientists who are making the miracle happen, we have a good chance of sharing the historic celebration that's coming. Perhaps we'll see you there.

Patrick is what used to be referred to as a polymath. He has a specialist's understanding of many subjects and, like all true polymaths, is largely self-taught. No topic is foreign to him. He sees all of them as neighborhoods spread across a single landscape.

He has proven he has a sharp eye for identifying transformational technologies, but it's not just talent. He works at it full time. He consumes medical journals and patent applications with all the gusto my family brings to Thanksgiving dinner. And he's wired in, having spent decades accumulating the private phone numbers and email addresses of the most brilliant and determined researchers, scientists, and investors in the biotech world.

I've seen the power of his broad knowledge. After digesting an arcane research report, he'll pick up the phone and alert the author to progress in another area that could help the author advance his work. He's a pollinator of progress with dozens of thankful scientists in his debt.

I remember one particularly poignant episode. A close friend called me about his son, an MIT graduate studying rocket science at Stanford. This 25-year-old wasn't content to be an earthbound genius; he wanted to go into space. But he had just been diagnosed with a particularly nasty form of brain glioma. My friend knew I was an investor in breakthrough biotechnology companies and was hoping I could point his son toward a cure.

So I called Patrick Cox, who told me about a private startup in West Covington, Kentucky, that was developing a promising new suite of cancer therapies—including a drug that could pierce the blood-brain barrier and attack gliomas. Patrick gave us the contact details, and within days I, my friend, and his son were on a plane to Cincinnati to meet with the principals.

By the time you read this, preparation for human trials on their broad-spectrum cancer treatment will be far along in preparation. Then after a year or so, we'll know whether their "bullet" for mass tumors can work as well in humans as it has in mice.

It's amazing that Patrick even knew about them. They are a

private company and in the world of biotechnology startups, one of the more obscure. But information on them was available if you knew how to dive deep enough, and apparently Patrick had not only done the dive, he understood why the company's drug was the best bet for my friend's son.

In fact, his explanation of how the drug works is both simpler and more precise than the company's own telling of the story. Patrick has a gift for unfolding complex biotech topics and spreading them out for his readers to see clearly and quickly.

He lets me tag along. Recently, we went to Sarasota, Florida, to visit the Roskamp Institute, the world's leading research facility for Alzheimer's disease. There we saw the effects of a newly identified nutraceutical that was given to mice afflicted with multiple sclerosis. It was astounding. The therapy reversed the disease.

Even more amazing was the nutraceutical's effectiveness for Alzheimer's. Animals in advanced stages of the disease recovered their ability to learn.

All good news, you might think. But there's some bad news. The substance, which hundreds of thousands of people once used to treat a variety of conditions, was withdrawn from sale because... according to the Alice-in-Wonderland logic of the FDA, it seems to work and therefore is a drug and therefore must not be offered to the general public until it has completed the FDA drug-trial process. Maybe sometime in the next decade, most people will be able to get it. Patrick's readers, myself included, don't intend to wait that long.

Another trip took us to a Minnesota hog butchery that had made room for a biotech startup. The firm is perfecting methods borrowed from the University of Minnesota for pulling a pig's heart cells away from the collagen scaffolding that holds them in place. What's left is an empty scaffolding, which can then be colonized with human heart cells that—with the aid of the structure—should grow into a human heart. This is truly cutting-edge, breakthrough technology.

The scientists we met were clearly excited about their work. Later, Patrick explained that the real power of what they were developing would come when they used the structure as an assembly device for rejuvenated stem cells—the kind produced by a process invented by Dr. Mike West of BioTime. And that is another tech story Patrick introduced me to.

After the introduction, I scheduled a two-hour meeting with Dr. West in Dallas. Those two hours turned into ten. We discovered that our personal and philosophical journeys were as similar as those of twins and that we shared the same passion for fighting aging. Which is convenient for me, because he is the world's leading expert on cell regeneration and rejuvenation.

Patrick, Mike West, and I are all about the same age—at or near 67.

10 years ago, Dr. West's forecast for solving the aging problem was 35 years. Now he says 25 years, so he seems to be on schedule.

Dr. West has been a prime mover in almost every major advance in stem cell research in the last 30 years. He led biotech's escape from dependence on embryonic stem cells by developing methods for generating pluripotent stem cells. Now he can take an ordinary cell from any human (no embryo is disturbed) and convert it into a stem cell that can be turned into almost any type of human tissue. He has already done this with 120 human tissue types, including heart, lung, liver, kidney, and cornea. And the resulting tissue is functionally very young—as young as that of a fetus.

I've seen the process. He harvested skin cells from Patrick's arm while we sat in a laboratory near San Francisco. Then, after a week or so of treatment in a chemical bath that switched on certain genes and switched off others, the cells emerged as pluripotent stem cells. Then, with a second stage of biochemical treatment, he turned the pluripotent cells into heart cells, put them in a petri dish, and let them grow. Six days later, they were beating! You can watch the video at https://youtu.be/xd8HmNFPUeU.

The next year, he did the same thing with my skin cells, and then did a full genome study of us both. He ran the results through one of his Israel-based subsidiaries against a database of every known genomic study that told us the good, the bad, and the ugly about our particular genome. In a few years, this will be standard operating procedure for everyone.

Recently, Patrick took me along on a trip to the Buck Institute, which is the world's premier anti-aging research operation. It is at the very center of everything that science is learning about aging and how to stop and eventually reverse it.

One of the exciting things we reviewed was the Buck Institute's work with rapamycin. It's been known for about 10 years that rapamycin has powerful anti-aging effects on mice. I've seen videos of old mice behaving like young ones. But the substance can have serious side effects.

The Buck Institute is studying rapamycin's mechanisms of action to determine which of them slow aging and which produce the unwanted side effects. By altering the rapamycin molecule one atom at a time, they are creating analogues of the molecule. The goal is to develop new compounds, or "rapalogs," that preserve the anti-aging power while eliminating the unwanted side effects.

Buck Institute researchers are also developing a nutraceutical we will be able to take as a daily pill to soften the negative effects of aging. It could be available by the end of this decade.

Patrick and I both take a short list of substances that new science has identified as critical for healthy longevity, and we are both in better shape than we have ever been. You're not supposed to be setting lifetime fitness records in your 60s. Maybe for me, it was because I haven't always been as serious about fitness as I am now—although in my 40s, I was pretty much a gym rat. But I'm in better shape today than I was then. And it's not only me, it's other people who are hanging with Patrick. He is revolutionizing—and I believe extending—the lives of his friends and readers.

Two years ago, I persuaded Patrick to join my publishing firm where he now writes a pair of newsletters. One is a free weekly report that keeps you up on the latest developments in anti-aging technology. And for serious investors, he writes the monthly *Transformational Technology Alert*, which is a must-read among biotech investors. I'm not quite certain how he does it, but it seems that every month he finds a new technology with the potential to transform our world in an amazing way.

Did you know there is a company that can tag every object as it leaves the production line with its own unique code—and do so at a cost of a tiny fraction of a penny? That would make it impossible to counterfeit anything—including designer shoes, computer chips, or dollar bills.

Worried about cirrhosis of the liver? The Zika virus? Any virus? Patrick has news for you.

What nutraceuticals should you be looking at for your own health? (No, not the fad stuff, the stuff with real science behind it.)

New drug delivery systems, companies that have found ways to counteract modern mankind's tendency toward obesity, drugs to cure multiple sclerosis, and drugs that can help healthy people become extraordinarily fit... Patrick has more news for you.

All these things are coming soon. And because I'm standing next to Patrick Cox, I'll be close to the front of the line when each one comes out.

Patrick talks about these and dozens of other things that are truly geewhiz, unbelievable, amazing, and seemingly science-fiction. But if you are looking in the right direction, you'll see them all happening right in front of your eyes. In the pages that follow, you are going to learn how all of this has become possible.

Congratulations. You are going to live a lot longer than you once expected, and you're going to be healthier than your parents ever imagined possible for someone your age. The future is coming through the door right now, and you get to live it.

John Mauldin is the founder of Mauldin Economics and a world-renowned financial writer of New York Times best-selling books including *Code Red*, *Bull's Eye Investing*, *Just One Thing*, *Endgame*, and most recently, *The Little Book of Bull's Eye Investing*.

Acknowledgments

I owe a huge debt of gratitude to so many people, a comprehensive list would be impractical. Of course, my immediate family deserves the most credit for accepting my intractable schedule and obsession with the subject matter of this book. John Mauldin, who allowed me the forum to spread news about the solutions science offers, has to be named as well. Without John's support and the power of his reputation, this book would not have been written.

Others contributed greatly to this project, compensating generously for my limitations. To name only a few, I thank Terry Coxon, the Maxwell Perkins of the financial publishing industry, as well as Shannara Johnson and Michelle Burgess.

Ultimately, however, I defer to the judgment of economist Joseph Schumpeter, who credited societal progress, which ought to be our shared goal, to innovators and risk-takers. The innovators are the scientists who decode the rules that govern physical reality and then invent the tools of civilization. Many claim credit for progress, including politicians and writers, but innovators, together with entrepreneurs and investors (Schumpeter's risk-takers), are most responsible for overcoming humanity's primordial challenges, even when confronting enmity and obstruction. These are the people to whom we all owe the most profound gratitude. They are also the people whom I rely on personally for what I know and do.

Patrick Cox, Marco Island, Florida, 2016

Part I:

How Longer Lives Are Changing Humanity

Chapter 1

Fewer Births, Longer Lives: Society's Aging Changes Everything

The world is on the brink of a demographic milestone. Since the beginning of recorded history, young children have outnumbered their elders. In about five years' time, however, the number of people aged 65 or older will outnumber children under age 5.

Driven by falling fertility rates and remarkable increases in life expectancy, population aging will continue, even accelerate. The number of people aged 65 or older is projected to grow from an estimated 524 million in 2010 to nearly 1.5 billion in 2050, with most of the increase in developing countries.
—*Global Health and Aging*, National Institute on Aging (NIA)

T he world is undergoing a transformation so profound and so sweeping that it will upset everything about the way we live. And this great change is starting in near silence, as though the historical behemoth striding toward us is coming on padded feet. The radically new future now approaching is so stealthy and so little noticed that all but a few would be puzzled by its name—the "Methuselah Effect."

It will redirect the entire course of human events in ways that future historians will compare to mankind's mastering of fire or the domestication of wheat, though few contemporary historians or sociologists have yet noticed what is happening right in front of them. I found almost no mention of this world-changing event when *Global Health and Aging* was published, nor have I heard anyone in public life acknowledge what is happening.

Driving the remaking of our world is a stark fact: *From here on out, every generation will be smaller than the one before it.* After 200,000 years of population growth, mankind's numbers are shrinking.

It can't be overstated how profound the impact of this reversal will be on all aspects of human society, including economics and finance. But what is the cause?

In a word—science. Driving the demographic transformation now sneaking up on the world is the longer lifespans that nearly three centuries of technological progress have given us. Beginning with the dawn of the Enlightenment, around the time of the American Revolution, the accumulation of scientific knowledge accelerated markedly, and that knowledge and the higher living standards it supported have enabled people to live longer and longer.

Since the 1840s, life expectancy in the US and elsewhere in the West has been rising by nearly three months every year, year after year. An American born in 1900 could be expected to survive to his mid-forties. Today, life expectancy for a newborn American is about 80.

Although much of the rest of the world is still far behind, it is now playing a winning game of catch-up. In Africa, Asia and South America, longevity now is increasing even more rapidly than in the US and Europe, as Western technologies for extending lives reach societies where, until quite recently, life was brutally short.

Increased longevity is not just an addendum to Mankind's story. It rewrites the story. The age profile of the world's population isn't merely shifting, it is inverting. Some demographers call it "the gray tsunami." Others describe it as "the age pyramid flipping." I call it a world turning upside down.

Through all of history up to now, there have almost always been more young people than old people. High birth rates coupled with high mortality rates assured that the young were always the largest segment of the population. This simple graph shows mankind's demographic pyramid for nearly the entirety of its existence.

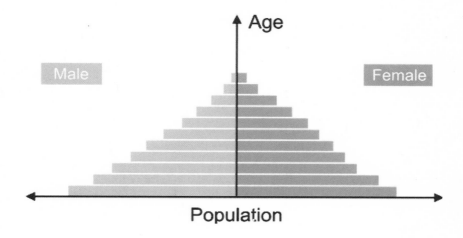

Trends that have been running since the late 1800s will draw a graph more like a pillar, or even turn the pyramid on its head. Population statistics are showing the shift already. In some still primitive regions, the old pyramid persists; elsewhere, most conspicuously in Japan, it is a picture of the past.

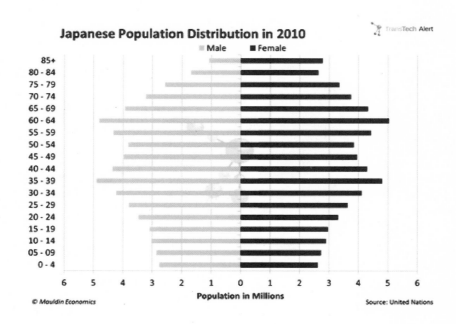

Today the United States' demographic chart is looking like a square-bottomed ice cream cone. And the shift toward a society full of old people isn't slowing down. In fact, it's beginning to kick into high gear.

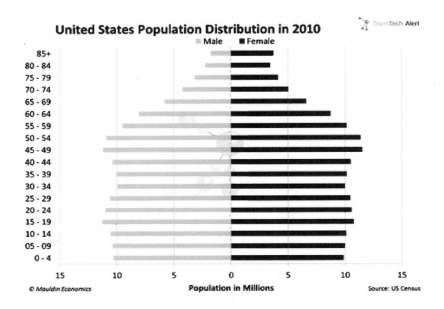

The shift is a grand disturber, but it is also something to celebrate. Despite all the criticism of the US healthcare industry, medical science has been astonishingly successful. In little over a century and a half, it has doubled the life expectancy of every newborn American. It is going to do much, much more. Hundredth birthdays are going to become unremarkable —and you'll see more of the celebrants actually blowing out all the candles.

The chart below compares survival rates for Americans born in 2006 with Americans born in 1901. In 1901, only about 45% of the population reached the age of 65. By 2006, the percentage of the population that survived to see 65 had nearly doubled.

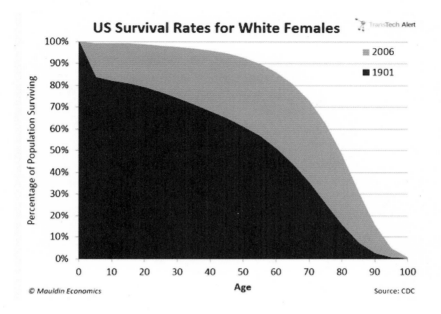

Chapter 2

Overpopulation—The Overly Big Fiction

For most Western economies, the largest single industry is conventional health care—delivering therapies that treat or prevent disease.

In the United States, health care accounts for more than 16% of GDP, which is significantly more than even the energy sector. You could say the business of extending the healthy portion of our life spans, or "health span," is the central endeavor of modern commerce.

Nevertheless, remarkably few people are aware of how successful this huge industry has been in getting the job done. Asked to name the biggest technological accomplishments of the 20th and 21st centuries, most would cite space flight or mobile phones or something else that is trivial by comparison with the success of medical science.

The true scope of modern medicine's achievement goes unrecognized by most because the plain facts are so far beyond the bounds of what seems plausible. In my experience, people generally react to any mention of "life extension" with skepticism and wariness, conflating it with science fiction and pseudoscientific health food claims.

They don't bother to weigh the facts because the idea of dramatically increasing the number of years we spend upright strikes them as a fantasy or a scam. While most understand that we're living significantly longer lives than our ancestors, their imaginations don't seem to have much room for further increases in longevity.

They should try a little harder. Not only are the trends that have extended life spans still at work, we are close to biotech breakthroughs that will accelerate those trends. The consequences will be far-reaching and in some respects nearly miraculous, although they will come with the social discomfort that always accompanies radical change.

In later chapters, I'll describe some of the technologies now emerging that will let you grow very old in very good health. These developments are not just theoretical, proposed or hoped for. They are well along the path toward practical application—yet are still largely unknown to the public. All in all, it is wonderful news, but each of the technologies carries social and financial implications that will be inconvenient for some.

Life extension technologies not only allow individuals to live healthier and longer lives, they are driving what may be the most profound cultural shift the human race has ever experienced. After millennia during which every aspect of society was conditioned by the general population's almost perpetual youth and its constantly growing numbers, mankind will be aging and its numbers will be shrinking. There will be fewer of us, and far fewer of us who are young.

The Forgotten Prophet

If it were just that people lived longer, populations would continue to grow, although on average they'd be older. But that's not all that is happening. Something else is at work. As lives have grown longer, birth rates have fallen.

There are competing theories as to why this pattern prevails in all societies where longevity is increasing, but prevail it does. As a result, as the number of older people is growing, the number of younger people is shrinking.

In most of the world, fertility rates have dropped well below the replacement rate (steady population size) of 2.1 lifetime births per female. Total populations in India and China and parts of Africa are still expanding and will continue to do so for a few decades, but not because there are so many births. It's because people are living longer.

When I speak in public about life-extending technologies, I'm always asked how we could possibly deal with the overpopulation that will result. I guess it shouldn't surprise me that some people still believe human populations are growing at a catastrophic rate. Overpopulation has been a mass media staple for decades. But it's a fiction, like Wolverine.

It's remarkable that the popular media have gotten away with it for so long. Demographers have been telling us for nearly a hundred years that the trend in play is toward a shrinking population because, as sociologist Warren Thompson observed in the 1920s, longer life spans are inevitably accompanied by falling birth rates.

In 1922, Thompson was hired by newspaper publisher Edward W. Scripps to run the world's first foundation for population research. From the data assembled for the foundation's work, he concluded that a profound change in human behavior happens whenever a society's longevity increases. He didn't try to account for the change, but he did document it, and he found no clear exceptions.

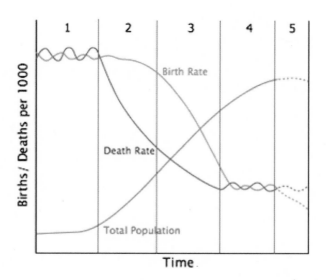

Source: Wikipedia

He called the consequences he foresaw the *demographic transition*, which was being driven by improved living conditions and health technology. As people lived longer, birth rates dropped. The arithmetic left little room for doubt. So as health and overall living conditions continued to improve, populations would stabilize and even begin to shrink.

It's hard to imagine today how revolutionary his work was. He was calmly announcing a break with all of human experience. His analysis predicted our current situation—the lowest birth rates and largest elder populations in history.

Thompson wasn't an obscure, think-tank hermit. Sponsorship by

Scripps assured that his findings would reach the public. And his book, *Population Problems*, became a standard university sociology text and remained so until the 1960s.

Then academia and the mass media fell in love with a fallacy—the Malthusian prediction of doom. Thompson slipped from the required reading lists, and entomologist Paul Ehrlich became a celebrity with his forecasts of catastrophic overpopulation and civilizational collapse.

Erlich has since been discredited, and the global famine he predicted is now long overdue. Nonetheless, Al Gore and others continue to hold on to the idea of overpopulation as a threat to humankind's existence. For some, Malthusian thinking is just too gratifying to give up.

Even Thompson himself found his conclusions difficult to accept completely. Having studied Japan, he doubted that the country, which prior to World War II had an extremely high birth rate, would undergo the same shift toward population decline as the rest of the developed world.

Today Japan's population is shrinking dramatically. Thompson only needed to wait.

In trying to understand Japan's stagnation since the early 1990s, economists have focused on everything but demographics. They overlook the obvious, crucial fact that the size of the Japanese work force is falling, while the number of seniors that those fewer workers must support continues to rise.

The Japanese government is fighting depopulation by offering tax and other incentives similar to those offered by governments in Sweden and Germany. However, in all three countries, birth rates are too low to prevent the population from shrinking.

Japan: The First Domino to Fall

In 1940, Japan's fertility rate, measured in lifetime births per female, was 4.1. The Japanese population was growing rapidly. Today Japan's fertility rate is 1.4… one of the lowest in the world and well below the replacement rate of 2.1 that keeps a population constant.

The impact is stark. Schools all over Japan now stand empty, and whole villages are populated by oldsters who seldom see children at all. In 2014, the Japanese population fell by 250,000, despite the country having one of the longest life expectancies. Japan now has fewer people under the age of 30 than over 30.

The Japanese recognize that they are in a demographic crisis. A recent Bloomberg article stated, "In 2014, aware of the dangers of becoming a nation of old folks, Prime Minister Shinzo Abe set aside 3 billion yen ($30 million) for programs aimed at boosting the birth rate, including matchmaking programs."

The same problem (too few young people to support a huge number of older people) is at the heart of the country's financial problems. This has put Japan in a quandary about two conflicting strategies:

- Encourage women to enter the work force to help generate tax revenue.
- Encourage women to have more children to provide manpower for future economic growth.

Japan stands out because the burden of caring for the elderly isn't just growing, it is becoming unbearable. But soon the world is going to see that Japan was never exceptional, it was just early. Many other nations are following closely behind, the US among them.

Flipping of the Demographic Pyramid

For a hundred years, anyone who investigated the topic dispassionately would have seen the likelihood that populations in developed countries were going to peak and then drop. Today the forecasts of Warren Thompson and other rational demographers are coming to pass, and native populations are declining at alarming rates.

The list of countries with birth rates already below the 2.1 replacement level includes Austria, Canada, Germany, Italy, Korea, Poland, Portugal, Russia, Spain, and Switzerland. In the US, the birth rate is close to the replacement level, but even here, the increase in longevity is pushing the worker-to-beneficiary ratio lower and lower.

In 1965, 9% of Americans were old enough to collect Social Security and the newly invented Medicare benefit. There were four workers to support each retired person. By 2014, the share of Americans 65 and older had risen to 14%, and there were fewer than three workers per beneficiary, hugely increasing the tax burden on the young.

Some countries, such as Canada, now rely on immigration to keep the total population stable, but that can't go on indefinitely. In many nations, like Korea, that once supplied immigrants to the West, average family size is shrinking rapidly. Many East Asian countries now have lifetime fertility rates of 1.5 or less, so their populations are declining.

Singapore pays middle-income couples more than $160,000 for having two children, but even that incentive has raised fertility rates only marginally—to a dismal 1.2 births per female. This means Singapore's native newborn population will decline by almost half in a single generation.

Even in Africa, birth rates are plummeting.

The United Nations, which at one time was promoting birth control to save the world from overcrowding, has accepted that population growth is coming to an end. A 2010 UN report, *World Population Prospect*, predicted that planet's population would max out at 10 billion.[1]

Researchers at the International Institute for Applied Systems Analysis (IIASA) are more emphatic. They calculate that *in a world with a fertility rate of 1.5, global population will drop to just one billion people by 2300—only one-eighth of current population*.

Economic Trouble

If people accustomed to worrying about overpopulation need something fresh to trouble their sleep, I suggest they turn to the puzzle of how fewer and fewer young people can possibly pay for generous transfer programs for more and more older people. If nothing intervenes, the demographic process now so conspicuous in Japan will lead the country to economic calamity and the breakdown of society. Then it will do the same in the rest of the developed world.

This is not a doomsday message, however. There is a solution. It lies in altering the implications of reaching age 70, 80, and 90. It lies in the emerging biotechnologies that will extend health spans, i.e., the robust and

---

1 See
http://www.un.org/en/development/desa/population/publications/pdf/trends/WPP2010/WPP2010_
Volume-I_Comprehensive-Tables.pdf

productive years of our lives. This will dramatically lower healthcare costs, extend working careers, and reduce the share of the population who are dependent on others to an untroubling few.

Media awareness of the emerging technologies and how they are going to change everything is close to nil. That seems regrettable but, in fact, is an opportunity. It positions smart investors to act on forces and trends few people have noticed.

Chapter 3

The Long View

From the time of Hellenistic Greece through the Middle Ages, life expectancy at birth was about 30 years. Average life spans crept up during that nearly 2,000-year span, but at rates so slow that, until the 18th century, the increase was barely noticeable. By the start of the 20th century, however, the increase was impossible not to notice.

Starting with the 18th century, most of the early increase in life expectancy came from better infant survival rates, which was the payoff from better nutrition, the germ theory, improved hygiene and cleaner water. Before then, only about 600 – 700 out of every 1,000 babies born would reach their first birthday. As of 20 years ago, survival rates for newborns in the developed world reached about 995 per 1,000 births, and then the rising trend leveled off. It had gone about as far as it could.[2] Most of the recent increase in life expectancy has come from better survival rates in each age group *after* infancy. And those survival rates keep improving.

The Personal Problem

Most people underestimate how long they are likely to walk the earth.

In 1992, a University of Michigan team asked 26,000 Americans over the age of 50 how long they expected to live. Nearly 24 years later, the Brookings Institution compared those expectations with what actually happened and found that most respondents had wildly underestimated their longevity.

---

2 There is, of course, no way to push the infant survival rate above 100%.

Big deal, you might say. Living longer than one expects is all good. Right?

Unfortunately, underestimating your life expectancy can lead to trouble. Most people seem to base their plans for retirement on their parents' longevity and leave themselves financially unprepared for their own, longer life spans.

Increasing Longevity + Entitlement Programs = US Government Bankruptcy

A 2014 white paper from the Brookings Institution[3] tacitly recognized that demographic change is at the root of the retirement planning problem. It acknowledged that life-extending technologies have fed the size of the aged population while falling birth rates are delivering only a dwindling pool of young workers to support the oldsters.

Today Social Security and Medicare—transfer payments from the young to the old—account for about one-third of all government spending, a share that has doubled during my lifetime. That share is still growing.

A 2011 report from the National Institute on Aging gives this warning:

> Some governments have begun to plan for the long term, but most have not. The window of opportunity for reform is closing fast as the pace of population aging accelerates. While Europe currently has four people of working age for every older person, it will have only two workers per older person by 2050. In some countries the share of gross domestic product devoted to social insurance for older people is expected to more than double in upcoming years. Countries therefore have only a few years to intensify efforts before demographic effects come to bear.[4]

The situation hasn't changed since the NIA report four years ago—except by becoming even more urgent. At some point, even in the United States, political willingness to honor promises made to seniors on the

---

3 *Better Financial Security in Retirement? Realizing the Promise of Longevity Annuities*
4 *Global Health and Aging*, National Institute on Aging (NIA)

campaign trail is going to succumb to the inability to do so.

The US government's growing indebtedness to its bondholders is a real problem, but it is still only the annoying mouse in the room. The elephant is the trillions of dollars in promises that have already been made to tomorrow's elderly. These are the "unfunded liabilities" that we hear about now and then (but only now and then).

A few years ago, *CNN Money* published, "National debt: Why entitlement spending must be reined in." The first few paragraphs stated:

> Medicare, Medicaid and Social Security are three of the government's most popular and relied-upon programs.
>
> So why does Congress need to curb the growth in spending on them?
>
> First answer: It's the biggest driver of the long-term national debt.
>
> Eliminate all the waste, fraud and abuse you can find. Cut even more out of discretionary programs, including defense. And tax the heck out of Warren Buffett and his pals. All those moves combined still won't do enough to rein in national debt.
>
> That's because they're not the main cause of long-term deficits. An aging population and rising healthcare costs are. So is the fact that there will be fewer workers per retiree paying taxes into the programs.

The article included a chart for one of those programs, Medicare.

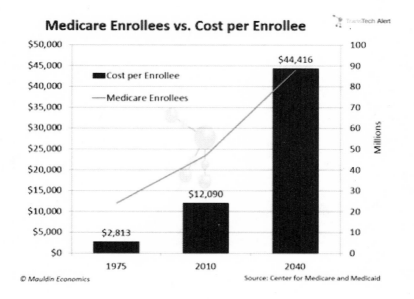

In 2014, the Heritage Foundation, using information provided by the Congressional Budget Office and Office of Management and Budget, projected that "all tax revenue will go toward entitlements and net interest by 2030."[5]

That means in just 15 years, every penny of taxpayer money will be needed for just three federal programs that serve the aging population.

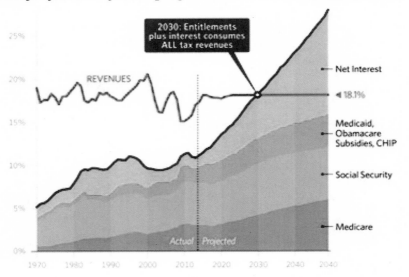

Should We Squeeze the Youngsters More?

The default strategy for supporting an aging population has been to make younger people pay more into Social Security and Medicare. It has worked so far, but the strategy is approaching its limits.

First, there is growing resistance among the young, perhaps because of the recent years of economic stagnation in the US.

Second, even without that resistance, the bill for supporting the retired elderly will keep growing and growing until the tax burden for paying the bill shuts down the economy.

So far, there has been no open rebellion against the younger generation's tax burden, but I believe it's coming. Younger workers who feel their future

5 *The 2014 Federal Budget in Pictures.* See http://www.heritage.org/federalbudget/pdf/2014/all-budget-chart-book-2014.pdf

is being sacrificed for the comfort of a wealthier but fading generation are voicing increasing resentment.[6]

The 2013 Federal Reserve Survey of Consumer Finances points out the huge difference in wealth between age groups. Average net worth in the under-35 group was $76,000, while in the 65–74 age group, it was $1.06 million.[7]

Even if younger, less wealthy people were agreeable to paying older, wealthier people's bills, the demographic transformation assures that eventually they wouldn't be able to carry the load.

Taxation Has Its Limits

Economic growth won't eliminate the problem. Yes, economic growth easily translates into rising tax revenues. But expecting an economy with a shrinking population of educated workers to grow rapidly is like hoping for a miracle.

Raising taxes or borrowing also are dead ends.

There are limits to what the government can collect in taxes. It can raise rates to any level it wants, but higher rates are a drag on productivity and at some point yield lower revenue. A tax take of 50% of what an economy produces is about the most any government has been able to extract without sending its economy into a death spiral of shrinking GDP and shrinking revenues.

Borrowing is also a dead end. It's just another way for government to tap what the economy is producing. If the economy isn't growing, government borrowing can't grow for long. And even if it could, a little reflection on the power of compound interest will tell you that paying for Social Security with borrowed money leads to government bankruptcy.

---

6 Polls by the Pew Research Center found that half of younger adults, aged 18–29, the so-called Millennials, want the federal government to focus its resources on the needs of younger people, while 59% of people aged 50—64 want those resources spent on older people. See http://www.pewsocialtrends.org/2012/12/20/the-big-generation-gap-at-the-polls-is-echoed-in-attitudes-on-budget-tradeoffs/

Half of Millennials, in fact, don't believe that Social Security will even exist when they reach retirement age. See http://iomechallenge.org/the-study/on-social-security/

7 See http://www.demos.org/blog/9/8/14/wealth-distributed-extremely-unevenly-within-every-age-group

It's difficult to overstate the impact of having a quarter of the US population retire just as the number of new entrants into the job force hits record lows... and it's getting worse.

"By 2056," a recent report from the Bureau of the Census, states, "the population 65 years and over is projected to become larger than the population under 18 years."

Current demographic trends are on track to create an unprecedented financial crisis. The good news, as I've already said, is that there is a solution, but it won't be coming from accountants, it will be coming from scientists.

Second Bankruptcy Vector

There is more to the government's financial problem than having to keep promises to more and more old people. The second vector is this: With existing healthcare technologies, costs *per capita* rise as people get older. This is yet another statistical truth that seems to elude policy makers, journalists and the public at large.

The following chart displays data from the Canadian Institute for Health Information and shows how medical spending increases as people age.

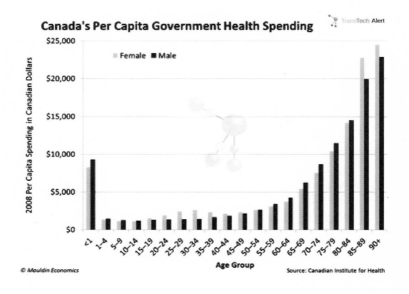

There's no doubt that healthcare spending has grown far faster than the rest of the economy in the US as well as in Canada as their populations have aged. Healthcare costs will always be higher for older people than for the young—so when society as a whole is aging, healthcare costs per capita rise.

Chapter 4

Demographic Tunnel Vision—America in Denial

S upporting a growing population of seniors is the biggest contributor to government debt—a stark fact that is politically unmentionable. Older people are a large and active voter group, which to politicians, means they are dangerous. They must be placated. So questions about the ultimately impossible cost of that placating are rarely touched on by politicians or by media cheerleaders for big government... which may be the reason the public is so little aware of the problem.

When polled about the government's rising expenditures for healthcare, the average citizen will cite higher prices for drugs and health insurance. In reality, increases in those two costs have lagged far behind increases in total healthcare costs. It is the growing number of elderly that has dominated the rise in health care costs.

Unfortunately, policy makers seem committed to ignoring the trend that explains everything. They prefer confronting the imaginary problem of overpopulation and its threat to the environment.

One notable exception to this see-nothing attitude is The National Institute on Aging, which published *Why Population Aging Matters: A Global Perspective.*[8]

The problems addressed in the report are not a matter of conjecture. They are already having measurable effects. Let me give you an example, the generally confused political topic of wealth disparity.

---

8 www.nia.nih.gov/sites/default/files/WPAM.pdf

Wealth and Age

Think about the fact of wealth disparity and then do a little arithmetic. The billionaires at one end of the spectrum are too few to have that much impact on measures of the distribution of wealth. Yet over the last decades, a wealth gap has indeed grown, but it is more between younger and older people than between "the 99% and the 1%." It is largely an artifact of life extension.

People tend to accumulate wealth through most of life. As we move through the stages of our lives, our earning power and our assets increase. If significant numbers of people earn and save longer, the wealth of older people, measured as a group, increases. This is pretty simple math... but judging by most discussions of wealth equality, math is hard.

It should be equally obvious that young people usually start near the bottom of the economic ladder in terms of income and assets. Most of us began our working careers barely able to pay our bills; typically, our assets were near zero.

That baseline is probably a permanent feature of the economic landscape. Even young people with advanced degrees and good jobs may be burdened with student debt, keeping their net worth near zero. The arrival of children makes asset accumulation even harder for the young.

The increase in life spans has left us with a larger number of older and therefore wealthier people, while the economic state of young people remains where it always has been. As a result, the difference in wealth between the two groups, young people at the start of their careers and an increasingly older and wealthier population, is growing.

How could it not?

Most Powerful Voting Bloc

Almost everyone in public life is covering his eyes, trying not to see the implications of an aging population.

Maybe opinion leaders simply haven't thought things through, or maybe aging is too unpleasant to think about. After all, old age is the prelude to death, a notion that seldom gets much of a welcome. Or maybe fans of redistributionist policies find it impolitic to tag aging as the real cause of the widening wealth gap.

In any case, the electoral logic of ignoring the implications of an aging population is simple. Older people tend to like government programs that send them checks or pay their bills. And on Election Day, old people show up, including old people who show up for little else. They vote at much higher rates than the general population.

As I mentioned before, as a voting bloc, seniors are feared by the people who live by election results. Politicians see the interests of seniors as a deadly third rail, and the rail's voltage is increasing as the number of seniors grows.

Here's some evidence. The next chart compares turnout for voters 65-and-older with the rest of the population. It doesn't so much reflect the attitudes of older people as it does the growth in the number of people reaching age 65 in relatively good health.

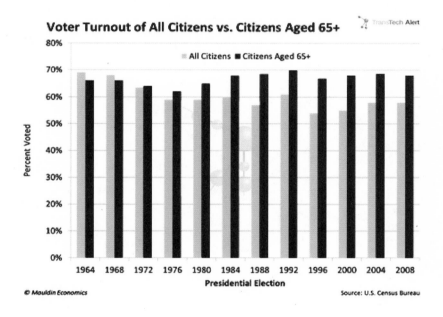

Fogies rule. And their hold on political power is tightening as their numbers grow.

So now the government is staggering under the cost of programs for older people. The burden will become even more crushing until it forces a change in mainstream thinking about how to deal with aging. But don't hold your breath. Even though science's power to control the effects of aging will continue to progress, I see little chance that the political classes are going to experience an epiphany any time soon. Until things get bad enough, they'll keep kicking the arithmetic down the road.

At some point, however, Stein's Law—if something can't go on forever, it will stop—takes over. The pool of younger workers will keep shrinking until it's too small to pay for all of today's programs for a growing population of old people. Then something will happen. The approach of government bankruptcy will force society to adapt to the new demographic reality. The least painful adaptation will be the healthcare/life extension paradigm being offered by modern biotechnology.

Chapter 5

Out with the Old, In with the New

C risis is inevitable, even beneficial in the long run. The business cycle theory of Austrian economist Joseph Schumpeter explains why.

Schumpeter posited that technological progress drives business cycles by undermining the stability of established institutions. For a while, the old institutions— which today would include Big Pharma, government regulators and bureaucracies and recipient populations—fight back. But the economic forces unleashed by innovation eventually prevail and destroy the old order.

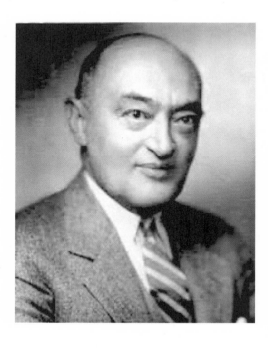

"The opening up of new markets, foreign or domestic, and the organizational development from the craft shop to such concerns as U.S. Steel illustrate the same process of industrial mutation—if I may use that biological term—that incessantly revolutionizes the economic structure from within, incessantly destroying the old one, incessantly creating a new one. This process of Creative Destruction is the essential fact about capitalism."
—Joseph Schumpeter, *Capitalism, Socialism and Democracy* (1942)

First-World Problems

The same technological progress that is extending healthy life spans will result in pockets of economic and policy upheaval. There will be casualties.

The trouble and pain needed to provoke a realistic response to population aging will be messy, but it won't be end-of-the-world trouble. I'm not a pessimist, not even about the near term. We'll learn and adapt as we always have. Today's troubles are easy compared with what the world suffered and survived during World War II and other calamities.

The future is actually very bright. The scientific progress that is forcing political and social change won't just extend our lives, it will enrich them. And as it is happening, biotechnologies that have been hindered by regulation and institutional inertia will be unshackled. Freedom will rescue the government's finances in a way that most people have never considered.

The pace of the technological progress that delivered today's abundance continues to accelerate, and mankind will adjust to it. The biggest adjustments will involve living without a constantly growing younger population.

The Waning Normal

As population growth fades, much of what we now assume to be normal fades with it, including population-driven economic growth.

All other things being equal, an expanding work force means a bigger economy. In the past, governments of market-based economies could grow their way out of financial problems, as high birth rates produced a growing population of taxpayers. As long as you could count on tomorrow's population and economy being bigger than today's—which was true for most of history—debt was manageable.

Those days are gone, probably forever. Growing populations will no longer be available to drive global economic growth. We've seen some of the results already in the sluggish growth rates in Japan and other countries undergoing aging and depopulation.

The following graph shows a 2008 UN projection of world population trends. Oddly, the UN demographers expected the fecundity of Western societies to rise to just below replacement rates, an increase that hasn't occurred. However, even if the UN's optimism about birth rates were correct, we'd still be on course for depopulation.

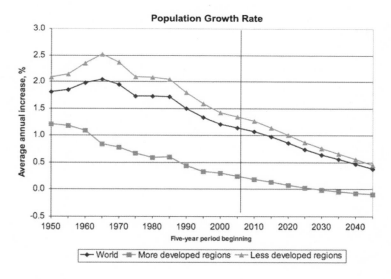

Source: https://www.learner.org/courses/envsci/unit/text.php?unit=5&secNum=4

The consequences are self-reinforcing. Pressed to support their aged, most developed countries today are eating into capital, which retards economic growth. Slow growth means less economic opportunity and lower income for younger people. Lower income for young people discourages family formation, which further accelerates depopulation.

We're already seeing this in Europe as some nations whose policies favor social welfare at the cost of innovation (such as France) are losing many of their best and brightest young people to emigration... making it even more difficult to sustain their welfare state policies.

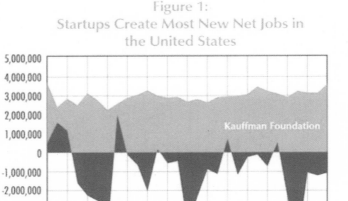

Figure 1:
Startups Create Most New Net Jobs in
the United States

Net Job Change – Startups
Net Job Change – Existing Firms

Source: Business Dynamics Statistics, Tim Kane

Of course, in some countries, authoritarian regimes will cling to the backwardness that promotes short life spans and high birth rates, but I suspect they slowly will fail. The dramatic improvement in wellbeing that began in the West three centuries ago, following the Enlightenment, will spread to most corners of the world, and as it does, the local populations will join the rest of mankind's communities in shrinking and aging.

If you don't know the work of Swedish medical doctor and statistician Hans Rosling, you should take a look. His video, *200 Countries, 200 Years, 4 Minutes*[9], puts the progress our species has enjoyed over the last centuries in perspective.

Even positive change, though, is hard. Many people applaud the reductions in birth rates and total populations, but adjusting to the new structure of society will present enormous challenges—in part because it's all happening so rapidly. From here on out, each generation will have fewer children than the one before it.

9 https://youtu.be/jbkSRLYSojo

Chapter 6

Baby Boomers and the New Healthcare Revolution

I t's easy to quantify changes in population makeup, but the consequences are full of unknowns. What's clear is that demographic changes gentler than what we are experiencing can have profound cultural impacts. You can be certain that something big is headed our way.

Here's an example of how demographic change leaves surprises on history's doorstep.

The war the Nazis launched in 1939 had a permanent impact on global demographics and therefore culture. When millions of male soldiers left home to fight, birth rates across much of the planet plunged and stayed low for six years.

Following the war, however, birth rates didn't simply revert to prior levels. They leapt, as though young people were compensating for lost time, and yielded the largest generational cohort in history: the baby boomers.

Impact of an Oversized Generation

The huge baby boomer generation has been shaking the world since the late 1950s. As this population bulge moved through society like an unbroken egg through a snake's body, it masked the fact that populations were preparing to decline.

The trend lines of depopulation were already in place before World War II. Birth rates in America began to fall before the war and resumed falling after the baby boom. The same happened throughout most of the developed world, but few noticed.

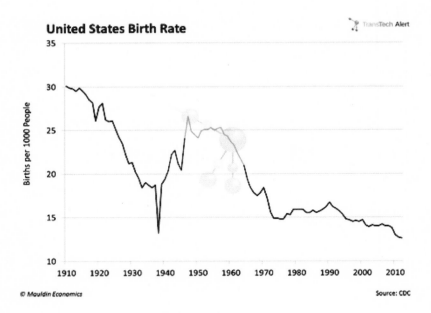

United States Birth Rate

Boomers were exceptional. Not only were they a throwback to a bygone era of much higher birth rates, they were a peer group book-ended by far fewer younger children and far fewer older children. That generational isolation opened the door to changes in culture. And as the baby boomers reached young adulthood, the counterculture they developed went mainstream. The world bent itself to boomer wants and boomer ways.

When boomers entered adult intellectual life, their numbers supported a peer group confidence that overwhelmed the attitudes and influence of groups older and younger than themselves. The effects still dominate in academia and in the media.

When the boomers began to have children of their own, the mass media turned its focus to child-rearing. Entirely new products, such as baby-carrying pouches, jogging strollers and computerized baby toys were invented and sold to boomer parents. When the boomers were approaching their peak career years, the mass media discovered career development as a topic that deserved more attention.

Now that the largest and wealthiest generation in the history of mankind is dealing with aging, you can count on society to turn to that issue. The title of P.J. O'Rourke's book stated the matter well: *Age and Guile Beat*

Youth, Innocence, and a Bad Haircut.

What will it mean for society as the ratio of the young to the old continues to shrink? Will children be valued even more than they are today, due to their scarcity? Will older people involve themselves more in the lives of the young, providing wealth and experience to benefit those with less of both? Or will society focus even more on comforting the elderly?

None of the answers are obvious, but I'm sure some of them will be less than pretty. I own property in Central Florida not far from the world's largest retirement community. It's home to 100,000 seniors, and I admit that I've been surprised by the behavior, and misbehavior, of older adults when their numbers are concentrated and kids are nowhere to be seen—from deadly levels of alcohol consumption to high rates of sexually transmitted disease.

Whenever I point this out, I get complaints, but I'm not picking on this community. I don't think any large group of older people would be much different, though I wonder what effect much longer lives will have on the survival of marriages.

They Still Want What They Want...
And They Want It Now

Because boomers are now older and slowing down somewhat, you might suspect that their influence is waning.

Speed, however, is overrated.

The boomers' wealth and political influence are greater than they've ever been, and boomers have more and more time on their hands. We just now are beginning to feel their full force. To anticipate the consequences, we should ask ourselves what baby boomers want now, since they've almost always had their way.

Like every generation before it, this cohort is starting to feel its own mortality. Old age seems to come as a surprise to everyone, and then the individuals who've reached it grow increasingly concerned with preserving and extending health and life.

This isn't special to boomers; it is a very old story. What's new is that biological science is now attacking the problem of aging... just as the oldest, largest, wealthiest and most pampered generation in history needs and is demanding a solution. As always, the boomers will be served.

Older people are already showing their irritation with the regulatory obstacles to better health, and the irritation is growing. Many leading biotech researchers are themselves aging boomers, and they feel the approach of their own senescence. They want to see their discoveries yield practical therapies… and soon.

Chapter 7

Adding Healthy Decades

T he growing urgency of the aging problem has stimulated interest in so-called "wellness." It's not a term I'm particularly happy with, since it suggests alternative therapies from promoters who are openly disdainful of science.

Nevertheless, the concept is sound. Maintaining good health through lifestyle and other practices is clearly a good thing. It's a modest but worthwhile step beyond the traditional healthcare model focused on treatment of disease.

The next steps won't be as easy as broccoli and bicycles. Science is pressing on, but the pharmaceutical and medical industries are as subject to inertia as any. And their inertia is enhanced by a sclerotic regulatory system with its own inertia and institutional interests.

The effect of all that hard-to-move resistance is huge and deplorable.

The Barrier

If you developed a simple compound that could delay the onset of age-related disease, you would be prohibited from bringing it to market. Period. Under the current international medical regulatory system, no drug can be sold legally until it has been proven effective in treating a specific disease. Aging and death are not diseases, so no matter what your research has proven, selling the drug would make you a criminal.

By the way, simple compounds capable of delaying the onset of accelerated aging in at least part of the population do exist. Some are already approved for specific disorders, such as ibuprofen, statins, rapamycin, lithium and growth hormone releasing hormone (GHRH).

Even more powerful anti-aging compounds have been discovered, but no company hoping to get them approved for distribution can do so without choosing a disease and then running clinical trials. The cost in money would be measured in tens of millions of dollars. The cost in time would be measured in years, perhaps more than a decade.

To become legally saleable, a drug must work its way through the four phases of the FDA's approval process.

Phase 0: give very low doses to humans to learn what the drug does in the body (the pharmacodynamics) and what the body does with the drug (the pharmacokinetics).

Phase 1: test for safety in healthy individuals to determine safe dosage ranges.

Phase 2: test larger groups to confirm the drug's safety and to determine whether the drug treats the target disease.

Phase 3: test even larger groups of people to confirm the results of Phases 1 and 2.

A plan for each phase must be approved by regulators beforehand, and since they're in no hurry, the process can take a decade. *Forbes* magazine calculated, based on the total cost of drug approval efforts divided by the number of actual approvals, that the cost per approval exceeds $4 billion. Moreover, the process has a **Phase 4**, which is the post-marketing monitoring of patients whose use the drug.

Red Tape Strangles People

By delaying effective therapies, the regulatory system causes far more suffering and death than it prevents with its focus on keeping bad drugs off the market.

Some scientists, including ex-FDA chief Dr. Andrew von Eschenbach, have called for bypassing Phase 2 and Phase 3 trials as a requirement for drug approval. Learn what the drug does in the body, test for safety and then go to market. Japan, which has come to grips with the need to speed therapies to market, has already shifted toward Eschenback's protocol.

In some notable cases, scientists who developed life-extension therapies with naturally occurring molecules are sidestepping the FDA approval process entirely by labeling their products as "nutraceuticals" rather than as "drugs." The distinction is a legal fiction, but avoiding the word "drug" can allow a naturally-occurring compound come to market without vast expense or years of delay.

A molecule that is found naturally in the human body is much less likely to be toxic than an invented molecule. The regulators seem to understand this, and there is a Washington lobby that tries to keep the FDA from forgetting the point. Shortening "time to market" is immensely important for a drug company. This has led to an increase in the number of potent over-the-counter molecules sold as supplements rather than drugs.

Naturally-occurring nicotinamide riboside (NR), which has been shown to reverse aging in animals, is a good example. Respected older scientists from major universities have stated plainly that because of their own need for effective anti-aging therapeutics, they would rather have access to NR today than wait for it to be approved by the FDA. If NR were legally classified as a drug candidate, it would be unavailable to them and to everybody else for many years.

In the case of another a drug candidate with anti-aging properties, the company that developed it is actually hiding data on animal life extension—not because the compound doesn't work, but because it works *too well* in delivering remarkable increases in health spans. Company management fears that the regulators would take disclosure of test results as an attempt to influence the drug approval process.

This situation won't last forever. Behind the scenes, nearly every scientist I've worked with in the last decade has voiced anger and frustration with the obstructionist system. Few will speak out publicly, for fear of making enemies in the agencies that control their fate. Today, however, we're seeing a few bold calls for a regulatory model based on "wellness" rather than on disease. While we're waiting for those calls to be answered, let's take a look at anti-aging products already making it to market.

Rehabbing Nutraceutical Molecules

The use of selected over-the-counter nutraceuticals—naturally occurring molecules—for slowing the aging process is now being endorsed by mainstream scientists from major universities, including a Nobel Prize winner. They have made it clear that they won't wait for regulatory approval to recommend use of these anti-aging compounds.

One of these compounds, which has the support of numerous academic institutions, increases *charged nicotinamide adenine dinucleotide (NAD+)* in humans. NAD+ is essential for the energy production that goes on constantly in every cell of your body. The amount present in each cell declines with age, which impairs all of the cell's functions. A compound that restores NAD+ to youthful levels has shown powerful anti-aging effects in both animals and people.

Instead of spending tens of millions of dollars and waiting a decade for FDA approval, the compound's developer plans to market it in a blend of molecules they believe will delay age-related diseases and prolong health spans. Most of the principals are about my age, the technical term for which is "old," so an FDA blessing would come too late to do them any good.

I personally have used the compound for several years. I'll give you more information about it in Part III, including how you can get it and what it can do for you.

The reason these anti-aging compounds can be sold and used now without government approval is that, being natural products, they don't fit the legal definition of "drug" under the Dietary Supplement Health and Education Act (DSHEA) of 1994. Other countries, including Japan, the UK and Canada, have similar laws exempting naturally occurring molecules, either extracted from a natural source or synthesized, from regulation as drugs.

Some nutraceuticals are tested in clinical trials, just as drugs are. Trial results are reported in language crafted to avoid making any claim about a substance's effectiveness against a particular disease. Making such a claim without approval from the regulatory authorities would be a crime.

Diamond Foods, a California food products company that specializes in marketing nuts, knows all about that. When they suggested that walnuts help prevent heart disease, the FDA gave the company the option to withdraw its "walnut drug" from the market (because per the FDA's definition, only drugs can be used in the prevention, mitigation or treatment of disease) or to remove all references to disease from its product labels and website.

That seems to me to violate the US Constitution's First Amendment, but I'm only a citizen, so how would I know?

I frequently encounter skepticism about the health benefits of naturally occurring compounds. I do sympathize with that skepticism. I know there has been plenty of over-promising and outright fraud in the natural-foods industry, so it's understandable that someone would conflate "naturally occurring" with the herbal placebos that occupy most of the shelf space in health food stores.

The reality, however, is very different. Many of the most important drugs regularly prescribed by physicians and distributed by Big Pharma originated with the study of molecules that occur naturally in plants and molds.

An extract of willow bark, for example, was used for centuries to ease pain. That was before the active element, acetylsalicylic acid, was synthesized in 1897 and labeled "aspirin." Today, biotechnology enables Big Pharma to screen the millions of other biologically active molecules that occur in plants, fungi and other organisms. GlaxoSmithKline, for example, operates a research program in China that investigates traditional nutraceuticals and folk medicines.

Nature is the best-stocked drugstore on the planet, and we're nowhere near finished taking a complete inventory. Even at this point, however, it is clear that nature is loaded with the real stuff. Often a pharmaceutical company will develop a synthetic variant of a naturally occurring molecule not because the invention is an improvement but solely to have something that can be patented.

Chapter 8

Aging as a Medical and Financial Problem

I n publishing or speaking for the record, a scientist is constrained by what he can prove with the data that's available.

The problem with the data about the life extension effects of drugs is that there's so little of it. You can't put 10,000 humans through double-blind, placebo-controlled life extension studies and watch how long it takes them to die, which is what would be needed to measure a molecule's life extension benefits the FDA way.

It's not even practical to enlist the help of our nearest relatives, the non-human primates. Their life spans are far too long for blind studies of sufficient sample size to be affordable. Rhesus monkeys can live to age 25. Chimpanzees reach 50.

It isn't that nothing is known. The problem is that the knowledge can't be fitted into the FDA testing model. A biologist who publicly extrapolated from the available data to what can be achieved with a particular nutraceutical would be risking his career. However, when scientists are chatting in a bar, with one or two pints of Guinness behind them, things are different. In private, many biologists agree that *we're going to see health spans increase by decades in the relatively near future*.

Longevity Dividend

Aging is the underlying cause of most disease. In fact, aging is *the* medical problem. With the exception of a few genetic disorders and communicable diseases, all disease derives from aging and the degradation of biological processes.

As our biological systems get older, they function less and less efficiently. With time, each deficit aggravates the others, and they eventually cascade into all the major killers: dementia, cardiovascular disease, cancers, type-2 diabetes, arthritis, hypertension, COPD, obesity-related conditions and even depression. Given the government's deep involvement in medical care for an aging population, it is these diseases that drive the growth in government spending and deficits.

Why is government debt out of control? Because every cell in your body is less functional today than it was yesterday.

"Articulating the Case for the Longevity Dividend," an article by gerontologist S. Jay Olshansky published in the *American Journal of Lifestyle Medicine* in 2014, makes this case eloquently.

> In the past century, the average duration of life of people living in developed countries rose by 30 years. Most of this gain was a result of advances in public health that saved the young by warding off communicable diseases. However, in the latter half of the 20th century, improvements in lifestyle modification and advances in biomedical technology enabled people at middle and older ages to experience extended lives. Thus, aging as we know it today is a new phenomenon—experienced by a small but rapidly growing segment of our world. As appealing as our longer lives may be, there was a price to pay for life extension—the rise of noncommunicable fatal and disabling diseases. It was a fair exchange, but now humanity is left with the difficult task of dealing with this Faustian trade. A new approach to public health in a rapidly aging world has been proposed (the longevity dividend), with the idea that extending healthy life by slowing aging may prove to be the most efficient way to combat the fatal and disabling diseases that plague us today. Here, I articulate the case for why we now need to turn our attention to combating aging itself.

The understanding of how biological systems degrade with age has increased enormously in just the last few years. We have reached the beginnings of the ability to slow aging—and even reverse it.

This progress is wonderful news, of course, but it is proceeding against a headwind.

The public seldom learns about innovative treatments until they've been approved by regulators, who seem to believe they are the only adults in the room. Usually, you hear about a new option only when your doctor tells you about it. Occasionally, a medical crisis, such as the recent Ebola outbreak, draws media coverage of experimental therapies, but even then the stories are framed to dramatize a problem, not to investigate the wisdom of allowing freer use of experimental therapies.

Things are going on in biochemistry labs that simply boggle the mind, but the most important breakthroughs generally stay hidden for years after the fact. For competitive reasons and sometimes for legal reasons, many leading scientists and biotech companies deliberately conceal what they've found.

My own work keeps me in touch with scientists on the cutting edge of transformational biotechnologies. Often I gain knowledge about a breakthrough only after pledging not to discuss it until some later date, such as when a patent application has been filed, which may mean holding my tongue for years.

A great deal is happening out of view. At this point there is a large inventory of good news waiting to be released to the public. However, while we wait, the transition to a predominantly older population is speeding up and the social pressure is building. It's approaching a point at which the rules will change to soften the need to keep advances in anti-aging technology under wraps.

Chapter 9

Progress, War and the Zombie Apocalypse

W e overlook how rapidly technologies change the world. The Wright brothers flew the first airplane in 1903, an event my grandmother read about as a young woman. Though the US military rejected the inventors' advice that aircraft might be useful in war, the first fighter planes appeared during World War I, a mere dozen years after the Wright brothers' proof of concept. Apollo 11 landed on the moon in 1969, just 66 years after the flight at Kitty Hawk.

Technological progress continues, even when everything else is going haywire. In fact, technological change seems to be fastest when things are at their worst. Look on war and other disorder as accelerators of scientific progress.

The Greatest Inventions Come out of Crises

Rather than slowing innovation, financial woes can accelerate it by increasing its value and sweeping away institutional resistance. The Great Depression was rich in technological breakthroughs, both theoretical and practical.

In the midst of the psychological and financial ruin of the early 1930s, home refrigerators appeared and quickly became commonplace. This happened not in spite of, but because of, the very hard times. The market for home refrigerators was driven by the need to stretch severely strained budgets. Refrigerators quickly turned from a luxury to a practical necessity because they paid for themselves by saving time and money for a population that needed more of both.

A fridge owner only needed a single shopping trip to stock up for several days of meals, which saved time and transportation costs. He could buy some items in bulk, at lower prices. Leftovers could be saved for another meal, instead of being fed to animals or tossed out. And using a refrigerator for food storage cut the incidence of food poisoning.

Applying refrigeration technology to air conditioning improved the livability of hot-climate areas. Florida, Texas and Southern California became more comfortable and hence more attractive for development.

This is the hallmark of a truly transformational technology: It not only improves life, it pays for itself by reducing other costs. Such breakthroughs are less common in times of plenty and calm.

And it was during the Depression that broadcasting came of age. The radio became a fixture of the American living room and then a part of the automobile; and its emergence changed commerce and society more than the recent emergence of the Internet. Two decades later, the television industry took radio's success during the Great Depression as a model for its own development.

The Great Depression was the economic cradle of synthetic materials such as neoprene and nylon and of vacuum tube technology.

When things appear darkest, financial opportunities may be at their peak. Companies now known as Motorola, Hewlett-Packard, Xerox, Unisys, and Texas Instruments were either born or came into their own during the Great Depression. Investors in these infant companies changed their own and their families' fortunes.

A similar acceleration in innovation took place in the difficult circumstances of World War II and gave us antibiotics and radar.

Having resigned myself to the inevitability of a transformational crisis of the sort Joseph Schumpeter described, I'm actually beginning to look forward to it all. I'd like to get it over with so we can move on to the world that will follow.

Let's talk about one of the most obvious and serious stressors pushing the system toward crisis and why eliminating it will benefit both you and the US Treasury.

Alzheimer's—the Zombie Disease

When I was younger, I spent a lot of time in libraries, cruising the crowded bookshelves for a title to pull me into a subject I didn't yet know existed. That's how I learned about Japanese culture and the significance of Gojira, which in English is Godzilla.

It seems that Godzilla, who first appeared in full form in the 1954 movie *Gojira*, was Japan's way of dealing with the emotional impact of the bombings of Hiroshima and Nagasaki. Through the fictional Godzilla, the Japanese compartmentalized and mastered the horrific experience of nuclear destruction. In the original Gojira movie, the monster was a product of American nuclear weapons testing, so the connection was direct and explicit.

The Japanese invented Godzilla, but they did not invent coping. Every culture produces shared tropes that symbolize and compartmentalize real threats. Vampires and werewolves long served that function in the West, although today they represent little worse than a really bad date. And in some recent tellings, they're sympathetic and even romantic figures.

Today the West faces only one monster capable of destroying the world: the zombie.

Zombies have been around since the 1932 movie, *White Zombie*, but those early stumblers were a different sort of creature. They were normal people who had been enslaved by a villain, a concept derived from Haitian mythology.

The modern zombie, a person who has been transformed into a mindless cannibal, usually by infection, evolved from the 1954 novel, *I Am Legend*, by Richard Matheson. As far as I know, this was the first time we contemplated through art a terrifying, personality-destroying disease that attacks without warning.

Filmmaker George Romero brought the concept to movie theaters in 1968 with *Night of the Living Dead*. Though the word zombie doesn't occur in the film, fans soon applied the term, and it carried into the sequels.

You have probably experienced, at least indirectly, an actual zombie incident.

Think about it: Do you know someone who seemingly lost his personality and mind and was left a husk with nothing inside but appetite and aggression? Do you know someone who devastated the lives of people he once loved? Don't think instantaneous transformation. Rather, think of a years-long slide into zombie oblivion.

I'm talking about Alzheimer's disease (AD).

If you chart the rise in the incidence of AD against the rise of the zombie myth's popularity, you'll see a striking correlation. Moreover, Alzheimer's does have an almost theatrical potential to destroy the families it visits.

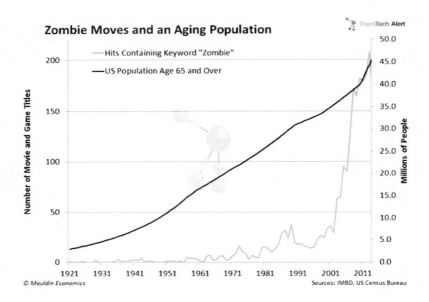

The singular transformation of the 20th century was the near-doubling of life spans in the West. Longer life spans are a good thing, of course, but there is a snake in the garden.

Diseases like smallpox and tuberculosis that once were common and life-threatening nearly vanished in the 20th century West. Antibiotics turned once-fatal diseases into treatable maladies. Even the old killers, heart disease and cancer, started declining, thanks to new therapeutics. People began to live much longer lives. As a result, the incidence of Alzheimer's increased, as did the level of horror it inflicts.

Not only does a formerly healthy individual lose memory and self when hit by AD, the lives of entire families are consumed by the slow devastation of a loved one.

Alzheimer's patients first lose the ability to remember little things.

Eventually they become delusional and lose all memory of those who love them and whom they once loved. Next, they lose motor function, moving very much like movie zombies, and, finally, they die, having drained the people who cared for them.

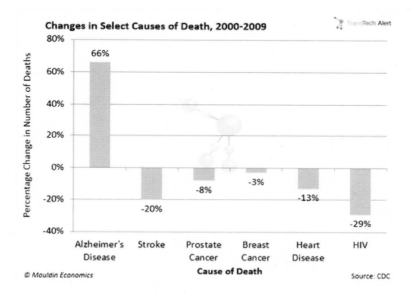

Unless your family has suffered this directly, you may not know that most AD victims reach a stage marked by hostility and anger. Nearly half of all Alzheimer's patients assault the people around them with hitting, scratching, grappling and biting. Sufferers of Alzheimer's disease literally turn into the aggressive zombies of George Romero.

Though AD is only the sixth-leading cause of mortality, it is this country's most expensive disease, due to the many years of disabled survival it allows the patient. Despite medical progress in most other areas, Alzheimer's and its costs continue to grow as the population ages. The zombie plague is growing.

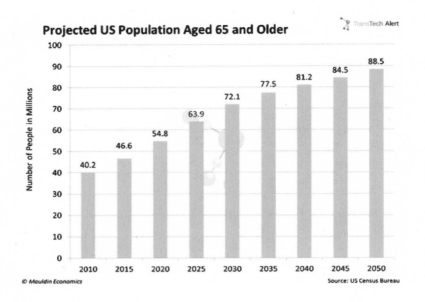

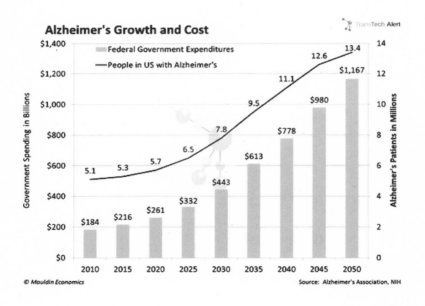

The numbers point to the real zombie apocalypse: Developed economies simply won't be able to bear the cost of Alzheimer's as the incidence continues to rise. Faced with an impossible financial, emotional and psychological burden, we would have to funnel so much of our resources into the care of Alzheimer's patients that the quality of life for everyone would plummet.

There is, however, an alternative.

Alzheimer's is not a simple disease, and despite some success in understanding and treating it, it's not likely that any single, simple pill is going to cure AD. Rather, Alzheimer's develops out of multiple factors—all associated with aging—that afflict individuals according to their genomes and histories.

The only plan for escaping the zombie apocalypse is as simple to formulate as it is ambitious: cure aging itself. To be more precise, the solution to Alzheimer's is to stop *accelerated* aging. We need to slow the degeneration that leads to Alzheimer's and other age-related disease.

Two social factors are at work to make this happen. One, the baby boomers want cures for accelerated aging. Two, the growing cost of Alzheimer's will force the politicians to get out of the way of the scientists who are working on those cures. What is brewing is a perfect storm of creative destruction, and it will blow away everything that opposes it.

Be ready.

Chapter 10

Telomeres and the Thread of Life

S o how long could you live, and what would your life be like, if we could put aging on a slow track? This is a critical question, and the answers will give you a glimpse of the medical technology due to arrive in the years ahead.

You began your existence as a single cell formed from your parents' gamete cells (sperm and ovum). The 23 pairs of chromosomes (long strands of DNA) in that single cell came one-half out of your mother and one-half out of your father.

About 30 hours later, the single cell divided into two cells and then the two divided into four and then the four into eight. At this stage, all your cells shared a remarkable characteristic. They were so-called *immortal cells*. It wasn't simply that they weren't showing any signs of wear and tear. Rather, they had not yet begun doing something that is fundamental to aging.

Each chromosome pair has the structure of a spiral zipper built of two long strands of DNA. When a cell divides, those two strands unzip all the way down to allow copying. It's an elegant molecular process that runs beautifully until it reaches the end of a DNA strand in a region called the *telomeres*.

At the very end of the telomeres, the replication (copying) stalls. The stub of the telomere region fails to be copied. This leaves each chromosome in the new cell with a slightly shortened telomere region.

During the early days of embryonic life, there is a mechanism that replaces the lost telomeric DNA. Each time a cell divides, a protein, called telomerase, rebuilds the small, fail-to-copy segment of the telomere region of each chromosome. Thus the new chromosome is buffed up to be a perfect, complete copy of the original.

If this telomere restoration process continued on indefinitely, a cell could fairly be called immortal. But it doesn't continue. Telomere restoration stops after the fourth day of embryonic life. From there on, each time a cell divides, the telomeres of the resulting cell are a little bit shorter. The accumulated loss of telomeric DNA eventually leads to cellular catastrophe.

By about age 29, a few of your cells have lost so much telomeric DNA (the telomeres have shortened so much) that the cells stop dividing—which means you lose some of your ability to replace old, damaged cells with new, healthy ones. As flawed but viable cells accumulate, you become less healthy and less vigorous. The early signs of aging arrive, and they never go away.[10]

The fundamental process of aging is the loss of telomeric DNA. Stop the loss of telomeric DNA, and you stop the process of aging.

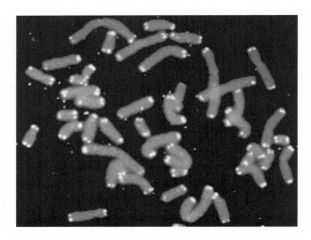

Human chromosomes. The white spots are telomeres. Source: Wikipedia.

In Greek mythology, the three Moirai (the three Fates) presided over the thread of each mortal life. Clotho spun the thread. Lachesis measured it. And Atropos ended the life by cutting the thread with her "abhorred shears." The myth spoke well. Now we know that the thread of life is spun from telomeres.

In your early life, cells in many tissues divide about once a year. Given their original length, if nothing interfered to speed things up, your dwindling

---

10 Also, there is a theory that long telomere chains move about the chromosomes, detecting flaws and triggering repair. As telomere chains shorten, this repair function deteriorates.

telomeres would stay long enough to get you to about age 120.

But something does interfere. Age-related disease puts your cells under stress, and so they wear out and must be replaced more frequently. The rate of cell replication increases—which is the same as saying that the telomere burn rate increases. That's why almost no one's life span extends all the way to 120 years.

Occasionally we read about a supercentenarian who does get close to age 120. What allowed him to approach that limit was the success of his cells in dodging stress and damage. It's the need to overcome cell damage that hurries the replication of cells and speeds up the spending of telomeres.

Hayflick Limit

The telomere budget set at the first days of life sets our maximum natural life span. Perfect health and a stop to accelerated aging would get almost anyone to age 120 and would get no one past it.

Dr. Leonard Hayflick discovered the finite lifespan of normal human cells in 1961 by observing that there is a limit to the number of times a cell can divide. It remained for Michael West and a company he founded, Geron, to prove that telomeres were the clockwork behind cell mortality. The maximum potential life span of normal human cells is now referred to as the *Hayflick Limit.*

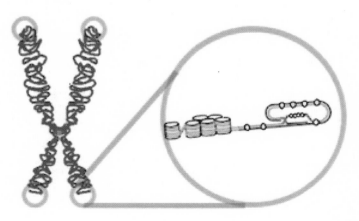

"Telomere," licensed under CC BY-SA 3.0 via Wikimedia Commons

Your earliest, embryonic cells didn't face a Hayflick Limit, because each time a stretch of telomere was lost in cell replication, telomerase would act to restore it. We'll return to this subject later because it is the basis of regenerative medicine and the prospect of living beyond the Hayflick limit of 120 years. But first, something a little less ambitious.

100 to 120—Supercentenarians and Super-Agers

When accelerated aging becomes preventable, life won't just be longer, lives will be more active and vigorous, and they'll rarely be touched by the catastrophic diseases that are currently breaking the bank.

This scenario is not mere hope. A great deal of research already focuses on two groups of people whose lives are remarkably free of disease—and of the medical bills that come with it.

The *super-agers* live in good health until age 100 or so and then deteriorate rapidly. They carry a characteristic variation of a particular gene, the CETP gene, and tend to have relatively high IQs.[11]

A second, somewhat better-known group is the *supercentenarians*. They live 110 to 120 years and remain active and vigorous until their last days. They seem immune to cancer, heart disease, dementia, diabetes, Parkinson's, and other serious disorders until the very end of their lives.

When time runs out, super-agers seem to get each of the diseases they'd been dodging all at once. Their death certificates usually include the phrase "natural causes." Their longevity isn't just personal good luck. Their families are spared the cost of lingering, debilitating diseases. Insurance companies and Medicare and other government programs save money as well.

Ironically, super-agers have good health despite, as a group, not having a particularly healthy lifestyle. Many drink, smoke and go without exercise. I suspect that their higher IQs aren't the result of higher innate intelligence. Rather, super-agers seem immune to dementia, so they keep learning throughout their long lives.

---

11 CETP is the gene for assembling Cholesterol-Ester Transfer Protein.

This is probably a bigger factor in adult intelligence than you might think. The biochemical circumstances leading to Alzheimer's and other dementias are present in people long before they become obvious. Subtle but significant impediments to learning may be building even without observable cognitive decline. Many older people develop strategies for dealing with memory lapses that effectively hide reduced cognition for years. If, however, adults continue to learn into their later years, they can become more intelligent.

We all get smarter as we age, but only up to a point. Then most people start having "senior moments," as if memory and focus necessarily deteriorate in later years. But necessity isn't part of the true picture. If not for accelerated aging, we would actually get better at thinking as we get older.

Research on super-agers has centered on Ashkenazi Jews, because many of them carry the characteristic variation of the CETP gene.

Oddly, I'm living proof of what that variation does. I carry it, and although I'm in my mid-sixties, I've never been treated for any major disease, despite having lived a non-exemplary and sometimes irresponsible lifestyle. I think my family know this, by the way, but I'd appreciate it if you didn't make a big deal of it in front of the kids.[12]

My own medical expenses have run higher than the average super-ager's due to the number of accidents I risked with cars, boats, skis and skateboards. In general, however, super-agers remain healthy much longer than the average person and spend much less on medical costs.

Among other benefits, this CETP gene variation maintains the healthy cholesterol and triglyceride levels of a child even into advanced age. This is why my cholesterol numbers are always perfect. I seem to be burger-proof. Somehow this translates into extreme resistance to cancer, cardiovascular disease, Alzheimer's, and other disorders.

The lesson from super-agers is that a simple genetic variance can make a huge difference in health. Not surprisingly, a large number of scientists are working to duplicate the effects of the gene variation. We now can synthesize the protein that the super-agers' CETP gene makes, and researchers are exploring how to use it.

Super-agers prove that death, while it still is inevitable, doesn't have to come nearly as soon as it usually does. Nor does it have to be preceded by

---

12 When the geneticists who analyzed my genome seemed to find the super-ager gene, they suspected they'd made a mistake. So they double-checked my DNA to confirm. Apparently, it's rare for anyone but an Ashkenazi to have this genetic characteristic.

years of suffering, frailty and high medical bills.

All at Once and Nothing First

When they do die, super-agers aren't done in by a single disease or organ failure. Rather, they come apart in much the same fashion as the horse cart in one of my favorite poems, Oliver Wendell Holmes, Sr.'s, *The Deacon's Masterpiece*.[13]

Here are a few relevant verses:

> First a shiver, and then a thrill,
> Then something decidedly like a spill,—
> And the parson was sitting upon a rock,
> At half-past nine by the meet'n'-house clock,—
> Just the hour of the Earthquake shock!
>
> —What do you think the parson found,
> When he got up and stared around?
> The poor old chaise in a heap or mound,
> As if it had been to the mill and ground!
> You see, of course, if you're not a dunce,
> How it went to pieces all at once,—
> All at once, and nothing first,—
> Just as bubbles do when they burst.

The poem is about a man, the titular deacon, who notices that carriages never wear out completely. Rather, it's some part that fails, making the "shay" or "chaise" unusable. So he builds a cart designed so that nothing fails... until everything fails.

The Deacon's Masterpiece is an allegory for aging. Few people ever wear out—they die of a single-part failure that sabotages the entire body. Just as we're frustrated when the failure of a single part wrecks an expensive machine, it often happens that a single disease of aging ends the life of someone who is otherwise healthy. Holmes was pointing out the need for medical practices that would treat aging rather than diseases, to forestall

---

13 Oliver Wendell Holmes was a brilliant medical scientist and physician and one of America's greatest poets. Many of his works are biological allegories.

such single-part failures.

Because super-agers seem to get every disease almost simultaneously near life's end, they go out fast. This characteristic, sometimes called *compression of morbidity*, makes it impractical to treat any single condition. So when we super-agers die, we do it on the cheap. You're welcome.

Replicating this mode of departure (as bubbles go when they burst) is the goal of anti-aging medicine. Recent breakthroughs in biotech tell me it's going to be fairly easy for medical science to make most of us super-agers.

Is that enough? Not a chance. A more ambitious goal is to emulate the health of supercentenarians, and I believe we can do it within the next few decades. Then, not much further down the road, I expect regenerative medicine to free us from the 120-year Hayflick Limit.

I have no doubt that many people alive today will live past 120. The only question is how much longer we have to survive to be among them. For those of us who are older, this is a big question, of course. But we are farther along toward the goal than you may realize.

Super-Aging: Cutting Healthcare Costs, Doubling Wealth

There's another, valuable benefit from slowing aging: Super-agers not only live longer, they have longer careers—more year of working, earning and building wealth. And being free of cognitive decline, they keep working well. Some work better and better, aided by their extended accumulation of experience.

If the super-ager medical profile predominated in the population, healthcare costs per capita would be less than half, maybe just a third, of their present level. And lifetime incomes would skyrocket because of the added years of productivity. The older you got, the richer you'd get.

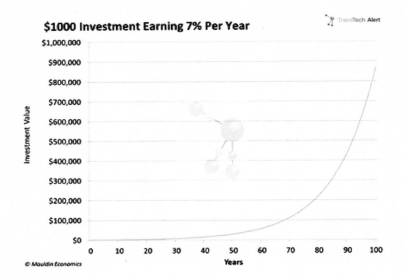

Chapter 11

Silicon Valley Kicks Sand...
At Big Pharma

E ven Big Pharma feels the rumbling of the shift that is coming.
With respected academics promoting therapies for longer health spans, Big Pharma is now moving into this not-quite-respectable area. And when the giant drug companies respond to the idea that healthy life extension is the only way to prevent societal collapse, research on the topic gains powerful protection from naysayers.

Big Pharma isn't the monolithic, homogenous culture the name suggests. The tent is so big that it can't help but cover a multitude of opinions and goals. Even different divisions of the same company may unknowingly operate at odds with one another. The industry is simply too sprawling to pull off an effective conspiracy.

That doesn't mean pharmaceutical companies don't have enormous wealth and influence. It does mean, however, that the wealthy left hand often doesn't know what the wealthy right hand is doing.

Many people in Big Pharma understand the threat of the "gray tsunami." They have projected the trend of Alzheimer's disease out three or four decades and see an unprecedented healthcare catastrophe in the making.

However, the guiding reason for Big Pharma to enter the anti-aging business is money. True life-extending therapeutics have been finding their way to market without Big Pharma's participation, and the industry is waking up to the risk of missing out on enormous profits from of life-extending drugs if it doesn't pick up the pace.

Convergence of IT and Biotech

Also pushing Big Pharma to move into anti-aging is the competitive heat from a new player in healthcare: Silicon Valley. The computer industry, particularly the big, established companies, have discovered biotech, and they want to own it.

The cultures of the two groups are entirely different. Big Pharma is a century-old industry manned by PhDs and long-schooled research biologists. It likes to prepare every move far in advance and runs business plans that assume decade-long campaigns for regulatory approvals.

Silicon Valley is another sort of people altogether. Many of the richest and most successful tech entrepreneurs were college drop-outs. Some never made it out of high school. Whereas pharma is slow, electronics from its earliest days has been the fastest-moving industry of all.

The winners in Silicon Valley have no experience with waiting for regulators to catch up. In the computer biz, plans are made and remade within days, rather than in months or years. The industry's hard chargers focus on immediate goals, and many will make big sacrifices to be the first to bring a new product to market.

Today, Silicon Valley entrepreneurs are supported by giant organizations manned with the best and the brightest. The one thing they're short on is patience. As info tech has matured, we've seen billionaires arise and pursue their interests with intelligence, nearly unlimited resources... and with urgency. Having acquired every toy imaginable, many top tech winners have turned their attention to solving the last crucial problem of their lives: aging. They know the clock is running out for them as well as everyone else.

If you know these people as I do, you'll have little doubt they are going to pursue their healthcare goals with the same energy and zeal that got them to the top of Silicon Valley.

In 2013, Google's Larry Page blogged about forming a biotech R&D company, Calico, and announced he was "tackling aging and illness." He went on to explain, "These issues affect us all—from the decreased mobility and mental agility that comes with age, to life-threatening diseases that exact a terrible physical and emotional toll on individuals and families. And while this is clearly a longer-term bet, we believe we can make good progress within reasonable timescales with the right goals and the right people."

Google is putting hundreds of millions of dollars into Calico and is funding other biotech ventures as well. Incidentally, Calico is also looking at ways to protect or promote NAD+ levels, as the nutraceuticals I've mentioned do.

Calico isn't the first Silicon Valley foray into biotech. Through his Ellison Medical Foundation, Larry Ellison, founder of software company Oracle, spends more than $40 million per year for research on age-related disease. "Death makes me very angry," the multibillionaire has said.

PayPal founder Peter Thiel, too, has spent millions of dollars on anti-aging research and awards grants to promising students willing to drop out of school to pursue their entrepreneurial vision.

While Thiel's strategy may seem counterproductive, it's not. Scientific progress is already far ahead of our ability to deploy what we've learned. Thiel understands that the efforts of talented business people are needed to turn the new knowledge into life-extending products and services that are packaged up and ready for the public to use.

Dmitry Itskov, the Russian Internet publishing baron, is focused on human immortality. While his vision of computer/human synthesis—cyborgs, if you like—seems quirky, I know that quirky sometimes finds the answer first.

Another notable Russian, Google co-founder Sergey Brin, is also pursuing anti-aging technologies. His most important life-extension projects are Google subsidiaries.

Smart Gadgets

Mobile health appliances, called mHealth devices, collect information on the functioning of the user's body and send it to a medical database, to make it easier and quicker for a doctor to identify disease in the user.

Virtual reality technology also will have a huge impact on healthcare. An Oculus Rift device can deliver tactile and motor feedback to the user. Such devices are already allowing surgeons to hone their skills by rehearsing high-risk operations in a virtual environment.

Other technologies allow doctors to retrieve information on the fly and expedite communication among healthcare providers. Fairly soon, nearly all medical knowledge will be available to nearly anyone. The experience of South Dakota rancher Tom Soukup illustrates how valuable this can be.

It was an old-fashioned kind of mishap: Soukup was badly injured by a cow. Unfortunately, the doctor at the nearby, small-town hospital lacked expertise in the kind of surgery Soukup needed. In a different era, Soukup's story might have ended with an obituary. Instead, his local doctor used video teleconferencing to consult with experts in a distant hospital, who guided him in saving Soukup's life.

Quick, easy sharing of information among experts worldwide will break down the borders now separating healthcare communities. Patients will have access to the very best medical knowledge, no matter where they are located.

MHealth includes watches that relay basics like pulse and temperature, but that's only the beginning. Technologies for collecting and transmitting more complex data, including respiratory function, blood pressure and insulin and nutrient levels, are in the works. MHealth will do even more to extend health spans when the data it gathers is integrated with a map of the user's genome.

Such systems would be helpful even if used for just one patient at a time. But much more will be gained by integrating information from millions of users into a shared data base—a new Silicon Valley specialty.

Genomics at Your Fingertips—Thanks to Google and Amazon

It's one thing to sequence a genome; hundreds of thousands of people have had that done already. To be truly useful, genome information must be quick and easy for scientists to access for study and analysis, which requires enormous computing power. The big tech players are now competing to host humanity's master database of genomes and develop software to analyze the data.

Of course, neither Google nor any other company is providing the server space and software for large-scale genomic data analysis out of the kindness of its corporate heart. The long game is to leverage the accumulating data into profitable new health knowledge by correlating the health experiences of millions of people with their genomes.

The discoveries that result will change medicine radically, especially by supporting individualized therapies. Personalized medicine has long been a holy grail of healthcare research. Genomics puts it within reach and will let medical professionals tailor treatments for each patient.

Google isn't the only high-tech player in this field. Amazon has its own genomics project, called 1000 Genomes. IBM, Microsoft, and others are also vying to profit from the explosion in genomic research.

Already, competition between Google and Amazon has driven down the price of genome data storage. Both companies now charge about $25 per year to store a complete, 100 gigabyte map of an individual's genome.

It's going to get much cheaper. When a person's genome is analyzed, the features that are typical of human genomes in general can be noted and stored in summary form. Storing just a person's variations from a typical genome requires only about 1 gigabyte, which scales the cost down to about 25 cents per year.

The science of interpreting genomes has already made enormous progress. Most people have heard that certain genes indicate a susceptibility to breast cancer, Parkinson's, and other diseases, but few know that it's now possible to use DNA from a crime scene to paint an image of the owner's face.

The sequencing and analysis of my own genome has already shown me how to live better. In the future, when even more is known about the impact of genetic variations, the benefits will be nearly incalculable.

Many drugs affect patients differently, based on their genomes, but we won't get the full benefit of this knowledge until the FDA allows us to. The FDA currently is keeping some extremely effective drugs completely off the market because they're dangerous for a small percentage of the population. The FDA doesn't seem ready to deal with the fact that those individuals could be identified by their genetic profiles.

High Stakes

Silicon Valley entrepreneurs know the enormity of what is to be gained from a new approach to healthcare, whether it's called wellness, anti-aging or life extension, and they have allies in the established healthcare industry. Scores of startups cooperate with leading universities on biotechnologies for extending health spans. Big Pharma is also in the mix.

One example is the Novartis Institutes for BioMedical Research (in Cambridge, Massachusetts), the research arm of the Swiss drug giant. It employs 6,000 people and is publicly committed to anti-aging research.

Novartis is reportedly moving an altered and patentable version of *rapamycin* toward clinical trials as an anti-aging therapeutic. The name rapamycin comes from the island where the drug was discovered, Easter Island, or Rapa Nui in the local Polynesian language. Right now, the naturally occurring anti-fungal made by bacteria is approved for immunosuppressive purposes. There's considerable evidence that it may extend health spans by delaying aging and age-related diseases like diabetes, heart disease and Alzheimer's.

Being a naturally occurring molecule, Rapamycin could have been sold as a nutraceutical. I suspect there are similar, perhaps even more effective bacterial anti-fungals waiting to be found by some intrepid biotechnologist. The tools to find them are widely available, and some of them are being used by amateur biohackers. Regardless, it would be good to see Novartis pave the regulatory way for other life extension drugs by getting rapamycin approved as an anti-aging therapeutic. In the meantime, a company associated with the prestigious Buck Institute for Research on Aging is moving improved forms of rapamycin toward clinical trials for various diseases.

Chapter 12

Health Tourism

An overhaul of the US regulatory system is inevitable, but progress in biotechnology is not going to wait for it to happen. As an American, I want my country to capture the wealth and jobs from biotech innovation. However, radical innovation *will* happen whether America leads it or not.

I regularly talk with executives and scientists who run cutting-edge biotech firms. Most privately admit their frustration with bureaucratic obstacles, and many have considered moving offshore. Some say that representatives of foreign countries hoping to promote their biotech industries have offered incentives for relocation.

More and more of the best US companies in my portfolio are taking their therapies offshore, where clinical trials are easier, cheaper and faster —but scientifically just as valid. Some focus their early efforts on getting therapies approved in Europe, a market bigger than the United States. (From a regulatory point of view, "Europe" includes Canada and Australia, by the way.)

Compared to the US, the regulation of medical devices is much more rational in other countries. In the UK, for example, medical-device testing has more or less been privatized, so biotech firms can shop among competing organizations for the best path to market. Once a device is approved in Europe, Phase 4 data from users of the device smooths the way toward US approval. Additionally, the UK makes many drugs easier for patients to get. Statins that have shown life-extending benefits, for example, are sold over the counter... no prescription needed.

Governments around the world have adopted a variety of policies to encourage clinics and hospitals that specialize in particular medical services—such as plastic surgery, heart surgery, or liver transplants—that are expensive elsewhere. Those lower costs attract patients who can travel internationally.

India, Thailand, Mexico, Singapore, Panama, Spain, Malaysia and Costa Rica are among the countries that aggressively cater to international health tourists. With much lower costs and medical outcomes that in many cases are statistically better than those of general-purpose hospitals in the US, they are globalizing medical care.

Health tourism has had a noticeable impact on smaller, less developed countries. Politicians and regulators, appreciating the revenue generated by these free-market institutions, approve cutting-edge technologies faster than the US and other red-tape countries. Critics claim this makes the facilities unsafe, but the data indicate otherwise.

Japan, I believe, stands to be the biggest winner in health tourism.

Japan recently changed its laws to cut the cost and time for regulatory approval of stem cell therapies. It makes sense that stem cell medicine would be first in line for deregulation. Unlike synthetic drugs, stem cells are a natural part of human biology, so we already know a lot about them. And the therapies that deregulation makes available will add to Japan's status as a health tourism destination.

The success of health tourism has been so pronounced that some medical professionals are considering parking hospital ships in international waters near New York, Miami or Los Angeles. Patients would be shuttled by helicopter or boat, without the cost and effort of international travel.

The availability of international alternatives is putting pressure on US regulators to move into the 21st century. The health and financial benefits of new biotechnologies will arrive, regardless of whether the FDA drags its feet. The biggest force for change is science itself, and it's pushing much harder than most people realize.

Chapter 13

Gigantic Progress on the Tiniest Scale

igh-speed computing has become a slingshot for progress in biotechnology. Today's faster computers (much faster than even a few years ago) make it practical for researchers to number-crunch their way to answers about complex biological processes.

And as computing is becoming faster, computer-driven lab equipment is becoming cheaper. Devices that a decade ago only governments and giant research organizations could afford are now within the reach of biotech startups, smaller universities, and private labs. Still cheaper and more powerful research tools become available every year.

Here's an example of how the slingshot works.

Knowing the exact shapes of proteins is an enormous aid to understanding what takes place in the human body on a molecular level. But gaining that knowledge, protein by protein, had been a nearly impossible task since scientists first appreciated how valuable the knowledge would be. Then research teams at Los Alamos, Lawrence Berkeley National Laboratory, Duke University, and Cambridge developed computer software that turns X-ray diffraction data about a protein molecule into a precise, three-dimensional image of the molecule. With high-speed computers, knowledge that scientists had been collecting a speck at a time can now be collected by the truckload, and it can be done quickly and cheaply.

Another example of computers helping with biotechnology comes from Cambrian Genomics, the first company to synthesize DNA with a technology similar to laser printing. They've cut the cost of producing custom-designed DNA by many orders of magnitude.

The company's strategy is a forehead slapper. Instead of using slow and expensive methods for synthesizing precise DNA sequences, they start with a cheap method for mass-producing a jumble of DNA at speeds of 100 strands per second. Next, they use their own computer software to identify the few strands in the jumble that have the desired DNA sequences. Any one of those just-right strands then can be accurately copied millions of times with an established, low-cost technology called polymerase chain reaction. The company is already using this approach to produce genetically engineered, glow-in-the-dark houseplants.

In the old days, investigation of potentially useful molecules relied on two technologies: *in vitro* experiments ("in glass") in laboratory equipment and *in vivo* experiments ("in the living") with living organisms.

Today, a third path is open—*in silico* simulation experiments, inside computers, that start with precise, computer-generated models of proteins. In cyberspace, scientists can experiment millions of times faster than in real-world tests and do so with absolute safety. For some questions, such as the exact choreography of the folding of a complex protein, computer simulation is the only way to find an answer.

As impressive as such inventions are, however, the fundamental reason biochemistry is now outpacing other areas of science ties back to the nature of life itself.

Nanotechnology: The Built and the Grown

A prominent goal of modern physics is molecularly precise manufacturing, which entails building materials and machines by manipulating molecules one at a time. We know this field as nanotechnology.

Molecularly precise manufacturing, which is still quite a ways off, will eventually produce submicroscopic machines, including robots, of tremendous power and sophistication. Materials will be stronger, cheaper, smarter and, like biological systems, self-repairing.

Much progress has already been made.

Nanotechnologists have built molecularly precise, microscopic mechanisms capable of performing simple functions such as movement under particular conditions. Given that they started with materials that are dead, this is an amazing feat.

Self-assembly (a fundamental ability of any biological system) is one of the key functions nanotechnologists are working toward. This is why carbon nanotubes, quantum dots and other quasi-crystalline structures are so useful for them. Under the right circumstances, molecular forces draw the atoms into useful alignments. At stake are results that seem to approach the magical – including nanomachines that could make repairs from inside the human body or turn raw materials into large objects, such as ships or skyscrapers complete with plumbing and wiring.

Though nanotechnologists tend not to like the term "nanobots," the expression is a staple of science fiction and the popular press. It's a good shorthand for nanotech's ultimate goal—nanomachines controlled and organized by a computer and reprogrammable to perform any task. While I'm quite sure we'll get there someday, that day remains a long way off.

Nature, however, is already full of such systems. Your body's power grid, for example, relies on trillions of bacteria-like, nano-scale mitochondria, each with its own computational DNA. Within each cell, the activity of several of these quasi-independent organelles is orchestrated by the cell's genome, and together they function as an intelligent network that responds to the cell's fluctuating energy needs. Everything your body does, from seeing to thumb-twiddling, depends on these natural nanobots.

Similarly, your immune system employs billions of cells that cooperate like highly-trained nano-defense forces. Some of them gather intelligence or information about threats to your body. Others store that information for both near-term and possible future uses. Some cells mark cells of interest so that other cells can easily find them. Some are attack cells designed for specific enemies, and others monitor conflict to call a halt to combat when the adversary is beaten. Others clean up the battlefield.

In the work of developing therapies to protect your health, biotechnologists aren't limited to the biomachines you were born with. They can draw from biological sources to enable your body to do things it otherwise wouldn't do or wouldn't do vigorously enough

Well Mannered Viruses

The term *biomachine* describes viruses well. They are as much a part of the world of machines as they are a part of the world of life. Like living things, they reproduce, although not by their own power but only by invading a cell and hijacking its genetic machinery. Yet unlike living things, they don't draw energy from an outside source. They straddle the worlds of living and non-living things and can be described accurately as naturally occurring nanomachines.

We may think of viruses as our enemies, and they certainly are. A single influenza strain killed 100 million people in 1918, about five percent of the human population at the time. And of course we all know about Ebola, HIV, and other lethal viruses.

Viruses are lean and specific in their operation. They carry no extra molecules. Some have as few as four protein-assembling genes, but they perform exact functions, eliciting specific actions that affect the organism they enter.

The narrowness of the range of operation of each strain of these invisible creatures makes their behavior predictable and reliable. Scientists are learning to exploit that reliability by genetically modifying viruses and turning them into nanobots capable of performing medically useful functions.

One application piggybacks on a virus's ability to insert itself into the DNA of a human cell. It is now possible, for example, to alter the genes of these genome hackers so that the virus will transform an adult human cell into something functionally similar to a non-aging, early embryonic cell.

A company I follow uses viruses to turn cells into controllable protein factories. It injects genetically engineered virus components into animals and people, to provoke their cells to produce desired proteins. One such virus component, which has been given to millions of animals of many species, enables the animals to maintain youthful growth hormone levels throughout their lives.

This virus-based treatment extends the health span of every mammalian species tested, in the process fighting age-related muscle loss, wrinkling of the skin, osteoporosis and obesity. The animals given this engineered virus are not only more fertile than their untreated cohort, they are smarter.

Think about the precision needed to turn a virus into a useful nanomachine. First, specific human genes able to synthesize desired proteins must be inserted into a deactivated virus. Then the modified virus must be slipped through the membrane of a human cell to deliver the protein-assembling genes. The remarkable field that makes this happen is too new to have an accepted label.

Killing Machines

A company that I'll describe later has built nanomachines that attract harmful viruses by electrochemical signaling and then destroy them. The machines are assembled by attaching natural components of mammalian cells to suitably shaped polymers. When a target virus docks with the natural component, it triggers an electrochemical signal that changes the polymers' shape to entangle the virus. It's a Venus Flytrap on an ultra-tiny scale. In the near future, we'll be able to treat virus-borne diseases easily and quickly using such bio-nanomachines and eliminate all symptoms of disease within hours.

Yet another company has learned how to prod brain cells to trigger the production of "search and destroy" macrophages that identify and remove accumulations of cellular junk that otherwise would degrade the brain cells' functioning. Though the macrophages aren't manmade, they are, in fact, biological machines that fit the description of nanobots perfectly. When they are activated, they immediately improve memory and cognition.

Each of these biotech mechanisms is in its own way a molecularly precise, self-assembling nanobot.[14]

Biological Toolbox

In the jargon of nanotechnology, the "wet path" refers to tools developed from DNA. The "dry path" is methods of molecularly precise manufacturing.

Nanotechnologists understand the power of biological self-assembly and the stark fact that DNA transcribes proteins vastly more complex than any object humans have ever built. So you should expect that, inevitably, the wet path and the dry path will converge

---

14 For some reason, the development of such mechanisms seldom gets the accolades and attention that purely synthetic nanotech receives for even marginal advances.

Think Big

Let's consider something a quadrillion times bigger than a gene: an orchid seed. Many seeds of the Orchidaceae family are less than 1/300th of an inch long and are visible only through a microscope.

Each tiny seed contains roughly the same number of protein-encoding genes as the human genome, as well as instructions for building and operating the elaborate biological machinery of an orchid plant.

While it may seem like a leap today, the tools are being developed to genetically engineer seeds with instructions for growing into almost anything, such as houses complete with matching furniture.

This is an idea that easily passes for science-fiction. But such power in a seed would be trivial compared to the miracle that turns a fertilized ovum into a homo sapiens. The human sperm cell is about 50 micrometers, even smaller than an invisible orchid seed. An ovum or human egg is about 30 times bigger, the only human cell big enough to be visible to the human eye, but the genetic machine in the nucleus of the cell is invisible even though a microscope. The combination of these two cells' DNA self-assembles into an organism capable of reading the words on this page and translating their meaning into actions that affect the physical world.

At the heart of all this power is, of course, DNA. Many scientists believe DNA is the optimal information storage, retrieval, and manufacturing system. Perhaps no man-made system will ever outperform it for compactness and power. The more we learn about our own biology, the more its own systems emerge as the answer to the toughest technological challenges.

This is not simply an ode to DNA. The most advanced robots and computers that have been built or are even contemplated are clunkers compared with the products of DNA. *Consider that your genome, which comprises over 3 billion base pairs, exists within each of the one hundred trillion cells of the human body... and every cell knows which genes to activate and which to leave idle.*

How does it all work? At this point, we understand only a little of it, but even that little has already led to therapies for many diseases. As the learning continues, the new knowledge will extend human health spans further and further.

Chapter 14

Action, Reaction, and the Shape of Things to Come

P eople easily accept changes that are small, slow and seemingly superficial. They generally resist rapid change, especially if they recognize it as radical. One way to resist is to ignore what's happening. In the foreword to the study I mentioned earlier, *Global Health and Aging*, the National Institute on Aging states:

> Despite the weight of scientific evidence, the significance of population aging and its global implications have yet to be fully appreciated. There is a need to raise awareness about not only global aging issues but also the importance of rigorous cross-national scientific research and policy dialogue that will help us address the challenges and opportunities of an aging world. Preparing financially for longer lives and finding ways to reduce aging-related disability should become national and global priorities. Experience shows that for nations, as for individuals, it is critical to address problems sooner rather than later. Waiting significantly increases the costs and difficulties of addressing these challenges.

That last paragraph understates the seriousness of the situation. You can expect the NIA's warnings to be widely ignored until there is no choice but to respond. However, this storm cloud has a silver lining. If you know even the broad outlines of what's happening, you can profit from the massive changes that will catch most people unaware.

Throughout most of history, the human life span was taken as a given. Increases were nearly imperceptible. Humanity's most important cultural institutions and attitudes developed over centuries marked by short lives, so I suppose it's no surprise that most people maintain attitudes that, though outdated, made sense for millennia.

The Bill for Old-Style Success

I hear again and again that an increase in healthcare spending as a percentage of gross domestic product (GDP), or total wealth, is a sign that something is wrong. Not so. It's proof that something is going wonderfully well.

Diseases once considered death sentences are now cured or managed. So people live longer. It is longevity, which proves that the healthcare industry has been successful, that has led to higher costs. It led there because improved longevity means more old people, and with conventional medicine old people require more care.

Young people don't rack up big medical bills. In the first third of life, people accrue about one-sixth of their lifetime medical costs. In the second third, they spend about one-third of their total medical expenditures. In the last third, they spend one-half of lifetime medical costs as they deal with problems like joint stiffness, failing vision, hypertension and, the biggie, Alzheimer's disease.

Healthcare's success will become increasingly expensive as long as healthcare means treating disease. Soon that growing success will become ruinously expensive—unless the strategy changes from treating disease to slowing the mechanisms of aging.

No one complains that we're spending more on computers, mobile devices, Internet service, or air travel than we did in the past. Modern medicine has undergone similarly dramatic improvements in the last decades. Unless we want to return to 1950s-style communications or medical care, costs will rise.

Yes, there are changes in public policy—the fabric of taxes, subsidy, and regulation—that by themselves could significantly lower healthcare costs. But not even the wisest such measures would come close to the air-pocket drop in costs achievable by extending health spans. Many of the biotech breakthroughs I'll discuss in Part III offer stunning solutions that are stunningly inexpensive.

The change away from managing disease and toward extending health will come sooner than you might expect. The demographic transformation will force the change, and the effects will be greater than all the medical advances from the Stone Age to today.

Look past the tangled problem of runaway medical costs and what you will find is the greatest opportunity of our lifetimes.

What We Can Look Forward To

Just in the last decade, biotechnologists have drastically changed their views of the fundamental causes of aging and disease. Though few scientists are willing to stick their necks out and predict publicly that we're on the verge of a leap in health spans, in private conversations I'm hearing this conviction more and more. Unnoticed by the public, a consensus is forming that the challenges of aging are beatable.

We are approaching a kind of biological singularity, which I think will arrive in two stages.

First, we'll see breakthroughs in understanding the mechanisms that accelerate aging in some people but not others.

We've already discussed the super-agers and also the supercentenarians, people who live to 100 or beyond with no more need for medical care than a 20-year-old. Their good fortune has profound implications for the rest of mankind, and we have already solved many of the problems that keep the rest of us from living similarly long lives.

We'll soon see decades added to health spans based on what's being learned about super-agers and supercentenarians. With the new therapies, healthcare costs will drop sharply because the most expensive disorders like dementia will be delayed into the relatively brief end-stage of life.

That's hard enough for many people to digest, but there is a prospect that is even more astounding.

Regenerative biotechnologies, or stem cell therapies, could extend health spans beyond those of supercentenarians. We'll break through the Hayflick Limit by reversing cellular aging.

A few years ago, such a statement deserved to be treated as science fiction, but a growing number of scientists in the field acknowledge that medicine is no longer limited to slowing the aging process. Technology enabling true cellular rejuvenation is now emerging. I'll go into more detail later, but imagine a world in which most people are chronologically very old yet biologically still young.

We're not talking about immortality, of course. There would still be limits to life spans, but they would be far more generous. Methuselah lived to the age of 969 years. Some of the people alive today may outdo him.

Biotech Hedge

While I didn't write this book just for investors, I think those who can afford to should join the class of people whom Joseph Schumpeter referred to as "risk takers."

Stocks of conventional healthcare companies are a hedge against economic downturn. Like energy and food, medical care is an essential, not a luxury. During hard times, it's one of the costs least likely to be deferred. Even during the so-called Great Recession, healthcare spending grew. But the big winners from what's coming won't be the established, conventional companies. The big winners will be found among the new, little companies that are focused on anti-aging therapies.

Any of the emerging biotech companies might fail—in fact, it's certain that many of them will. Innovation is risky, but the new biotech industry as a whole will be a gigantic financial success. Its healthcare innovations will cure previously untreatable conditions and, as a bonus, add to the customers' earning years. And it will be happening at the same time that the oldest, wealthiest, and most politically powerful generation in history needs it.

Preparing for the New World

I've been privileged to have a backstage pass to the show. For many years now, I've tracked down and reported many of the most important scientific breakthroughs of our time. I've been tutored on emerging technologies by renowned scientists in the biotech space, including Nobel laureates.

At the same time, I've seen growing excitement and optimism. But recognizing technologies that truly are transformational isn't simple, and the science can be confusing. The bigger problem, however, has to do with human psychology. In the next part of this book, we'll look at the history of disruptive biotechnology to learn what patterns of response to expect as the science of life extension disturbs everything.

PART II

Biotech Breakthroughs and Social Reaction

Chapter 15

A New Dawn for Mankind: The Age of Reason

E very era is modern... until it's the past. Human beings tend to see the age they live in as a unique culmination of what came before, forever dividing history into two distinct epochs.

The sense that we live at the moment in history when everything has fundamentally changed is probably a necessary feature of human psychology. Being alive does imbue the present with a unique importance. But since the dawn of the Age of Enlightenment, people in every generation have viewed themselves as unalterably modern, and this sense that we live at the apex of progress has only been reinforced by the acceleration of science and technology.

Progress can be confusing, especially for older people. In his 1970 book, *Future Shock*, Alvin Toffler posits that rapid change can psychologically overwhelm whole societies and breed anxiety and confusion. Nonetheless, there will always be individuals who learn eagerly and adapt to progress that is unsettling for others.

Cultural historians generally characterize the Enlightenment as a philosophical and political movement, but at its heart it was a scientific revolution. Its tenets, best laid out by the father of empiricism, Francis Bacon, led to a formalized, evidence-based process of scientific investigation that became known as Natural Philosophy. Though Bacon predated the Enlightenment, he paved the way for Isaac Newton's seminal 1687 work, *The Principia: Mathematical Principles of Natural Philosophy*. Newton, I think, best personifies the flowering of this era.

In the 17th century, "natural" didn't carry its current meanings, such as "not synthetic" or "pesticide-free." Rather, it referred to laws that govern all aspects of the material universe. Natural philosophers sought to understand those natural laws and to codify them as principles of physics, chemistry, biology, and others of what are now called the hard sciences.

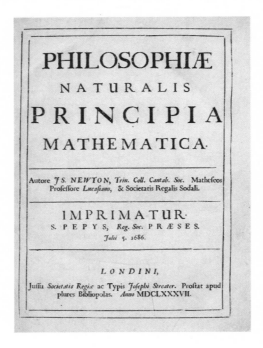

From Natural Law to Scientific Progress

As self-evident as it may seem today, the idea that the natural world adheres to permanent, unbreakable rules was quite controversial in an era when monarchs and pontiffs claimed authority over everything. The notion that natural laws cannot be altered or overridden by the decrees of any human being seemed threatening at the time and still does in some cultures that survive little changed to this day.

It wasn't Newton or other Enlightenment philosophers who introduced the concept of universal natural laws, though. Aristotle, Pythagoras, and other Greek philosophers taught that the natural world is governed by immutable principles. Enlightenment thinkers expanded on that concept and applied it to political philosophy as well as to the sciences.

In the Enlightenment, for the first time since the collapse of the Roman

Empire, Westerners who puzzled out the secrets of astronomy, chemistry, and biology received a modicum of respect and even status. In the centuries prior, tinkerers in natural law attracted the label of "alchemist," a stigma conflated with astrology and sorcery. Isaac Newton straddled the two eras and delved into questions raised by both natural philosophers and alchemists. But eventually he was made *Sir* Isaac Newton.

Chronocentricism: We're the Smartest Ever

Once people accepted the inescapability of natural laws established by God, rather than by human authority, they were ripe for the concept of human rights that exist prior to any human decree. Just as the laws of gravity and motion are independent of human authority, so were certain rights of people—a thought that revolutionized the relationship of government to the governed.

The practical consequences of this thinking were enormous. When combined with a new respect for science, property rights and their corollary, free markets, served as an accelerator for technological progress. Especially in the British Empire and Western Europe, innovation became rapid enough to be noticed within the span of a single lifetime—which was an utterly new experience in human history.

Today innovation is non-stop, altering everything from healthcare to food delivery to car design to home construction—and doing so as we watch. The transformations wrought by computers and the Internet heighten our sense that we live at the apex of history… but my grandparents felt the same way when telephones and then automobiles arrived and then aviation.

In 1969, after watching the television coverage of the Apollo 11 Moon landing, my grandmother told me how excited she had felt as a young girl reading the newspaper accounts of the Wright brothers' first flight, in 1903, before even the age of radio. The generation before hers was equally awed by the telegraph and intercontinental railways. Before that, there was the wondrous new world of steam power.

Of course, compared to nuclear and modern solar energy, Watt's steam engine seems clunky. Next to a smart phone, the telegraph seems like a toy. It's tempting to think we've somehow reached a summit today, setting our world apart from a past filled with error and naïve misunderstanding. We expect more change to come, but it's easy to believe we've pretty much got things figured out, unlike our befuddled ancestors.

I call this attitude *chronocentricism*. It's not that new. A careful reading of history finds that the attitude has been with us for centuries, encouraged by science's repeated success at overturning yesterday's strongly held beliefs. That winning streak isn't over. You should assume that many of today's "truths" will be proven untrue—even deeply held beliefs will be deep-sixed.

In just the last few decades, for example, the myths of peak oil and overpopulation unraveled. Practically everything nutritionists were saying about healthy eating a generation ago has been thrown out.

Moreover, we can't know what's coming next. The truly important discoveries arrive unexpectedly. Some of the most valuable knowledge that will emerge in the coming decade will answer questions no one has yet asked.

Scientific knowledge and technology are progressing at an astounding pace, propelled in large part by advances in computing technologies, but human beings are essentially the same as they've always been. Our current era will soon be viewed in the same way we now perceive the steam-powered 1800s.

Bottom line: We need to understand that although innovation is speeding up, our species' ability to adapt to radical scientific progress isn't going to improve in the least bit. So we should look to the past to understand and predict how people will greet the important biotech breakthroughs soon to come. By understanding the social response to transformational technologies, we'll be able to recognize and exploit the financial opportunities waiting in today's scientific progress.

Healthy vs. Barren Skepticism

My father was a man of significant accomplishment, a civil engineer who won design awards for highways and bridges while pioneering computerized methods of infrastructure analysis and planning. Not coincidentally, this was at about the same time that Sam Walton implemented similar communication and inventory control methods for his chain of retail stores.

After World War II, Dad parlayed his engineering degree into a computer programming job in the aerospace industry. Though he loved computers and software, he had no use for the cost-plus waste of the military-industrial complex, so he moved on.

In time, he got the engineering job he wanted with the Idaho State Highway Department and began moving up the ranks to eventually run the agency. His experience programming mainframes, however, stuck with him. When IBM started producing machines suitable for what he wanted to do for the Highway Department, he arranged for a purchase and developed first-of-its-kind software in-house.

I remember from a dinner table conversation that many of his best programmers weren't trained engineers but had been recruited from the women of the secretarial pool. I'm glad I paid attention. The lesson is simple and invaluable. In any endeavor driven by radical innovation, expect many of the best performers to be people who are short on credentials.

Chapter 16

The Antibiotic Transformation

Years ago, during a visit to my grandparents' farm, my father pointed out a sharp turn in a dirt wagon path where about 40 years earlier a horse pulling his wagon had launched into a full gallop. Only a boy at the time, my father knew he'd be unable to rein in the animal and that the wagon would flip at the turn. So just before the bend, he jumped, rolled through cornstalks, and landed unhurt.

It was many years after hearing the story that the real point dawned on me. Reading about the history of antibiotics, I learned that before penicillin, anyone who suffered an open fracture (a broken bone puncturing the skin) had only a 50/50 chance of survival. Because I had grown up in a time when the infections that open fractures invite were readily controlled by penicillin or other antibiotics, I hadn't grasped the danger my father had faced early in his life.

At the time he was born, in 1919, farm and industrial accidents commonly led to fatal infections. Until the closing days of World War II, dog bites were life-threatening, and simple kitchen mishaps left many men widowers. Then, in 1945, large-scale production of penicillin changed everything. Medical historians estimate that at least ten years of the increased life spans we enjoy today are due to the antibiotic revolution.

Fleming's Big Discovery

In 1928, Scottish biologist Alexander Fleming was investigating staphylococcus bacteria, culprits in food poisoning, non-healing wounds, and other disorders. He used dozens of lab dishes to grow cultures of the bacteria for study. On one occasion, before leaving on vacation with his family, he stacked the dishes on a bench in the corner of his laboratory, expecting them to develop thriving populations of staphylococci. Upon his return, he was disappointed to find some of the cultures contaminated with a fungus that apparently was killing the staph bacteria. We now know that the "problem" was a mold from the penicillium genus.

In one telling of the story, Fleming dropped the contaminated culture dishes into a sink of soapy water, intending to wash and sterilize them and restart the growing of the bacteria he needed. Only at the last minute did he realize he might have stumbled onto something useful and plucked the sole remaining dish with live penicillin mold from the soapy water.

Years later, Fleming said, "When I woke up just after dawn on September 28, 1928, I certainly didn't plan to revolutionize all medicine by discovering the world's first antibiotic, or bacteria killer, but I suppose that was exactly what I did."

Actually, we know that his understanding of what happened wasn't correct. The part about the soapy water may be true, but the notion that Fleming was the first to discover the mold's antibacterial properties is not. He was merely the first to get the world to pay attention to what others had discovered more than half a century earlier.

Not that he was playing loose with the truth—he simply didn't know that even before his breakthrough, many other scientists had known about the antibiotic mold. Papers had been published and experiments performed, at least one in front of an eminent scientific organization, but the medical community either didn't believe the results or missed their importance. Unfortunately, that dumb skepticism left millions of people to die of infections.

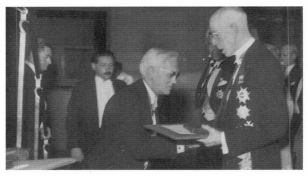

Sir Alexander Fleming receiving the Nobel Prize from King Gustaf V of Sweden.
(Source: National WW II Museum, New Orleans)

From Fleming's accidental discovery in 1928, it was only sixteen years until penicillin was being mass-produced for the Allied military during World War II. Just one year later, in 1945, Fleming accepted the Nobel Prize in Medicine. No one can detract from the accomplishments of Fleming and his colleagues, but we should understand that scientists had been trying to convince the medical establishment of the importance of penicillium molds since the 1870s.

English surgeon Joseph Lister (after whom Listerine is named) wrote about the antibacterial properties of penicillium mold in 1871. Though his writing gained little notice, he did succeed in using the antibiotic mold to treat the wounds of his own staff. Given the production difficulties encountered by those who scaled up from Fleming's lab work, that's quite remarkable.

Lister was the father of antisepsis, or antiseptic surgery. He developed and introduced phenol, then called carbolic acid, for cleaning wounds and sterilizing surgical instruments. His expression in this portrait betrays the attitude of a man well acquainted with the counterproductive skepticism of his peers.

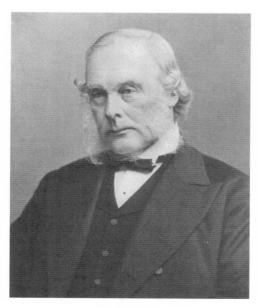

Joseph Lister
(S ource: Wikipedia)

Lister wasn't the only one to notice penicillin before Fleming. In 1875, Irish physicist John Tyndall demonstrated the antibiotic properties of penicillium fungus to the Royal Society. Even this renowned organization, however, did not grasp the importance of the discovery. Other scientists, including Louis Pasteur, struggled to awaken the scientific community to the potential of antibiotics, but not until five decades later did Alexander Fleming succeed.

Chapter 17

Fathers of Antisepsis

Lister and Tyndall failed to overcome resistance to what is now known as the germ theory, the once revolutionary proposition that some diseases are caused by propagating microorganisms. They weren't alone in knowing but failing to be heard. Others argued the same case, which was often dismissed by intellectuals as an unscientific belief in invisible supernatural forces akin to ghosts and evil spirits.

One important proponent of the germ theory was Oliver Wendell Holmes Sr., already noted in Part I. Remembered today mostly for his poetry, Holmes helped introduce the stethoscope and microscope to American medicine and was a crusader for evidence-based therapies. He lectured widely on the faulty reasoning behind common medical practices, such as bloodletting, and warned against mistaking a placebo effect for medical efficacy.

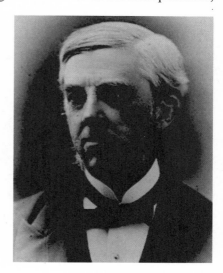

Oliver Wendell Holmes Sr.
(Source: The Atlantic)

Today the germ theory is so taken for granted that it's difficult to imagine that the idea of communicability was widely rejected in the 1840s, when Holmes was doing his research. Holmes criticized hygienic conditions in American clinics and hospitals. But at the time, many doctors resented suggestions to wash their hands or change their clothes between patients. Indeed, surgical aprons marked with blood and other residue were worn proudly throughout the day as a badge of the physician's profession.

An astute observer, Holmes noticed how common it was for a doctor performing an autopsy to contract the very illness responsible for the cadaver. He also documented clusters of lethal infections in birthing hospitals among women who had been treated by the same doctor.

At the time, such infections were called puerperal or childbed fever and killed as many as one in three stricken mothers. Holmes put forth his findings in an 1843 article titled "The Contagiousness of Puerperal Fever" for the *New England Quarterly Journal of Medicine and Surgery*. He theorized that puerperal fever was spread by physicians, and he recommended that surgical instruments used on infected patients be sterilized and that exposed clothing be burned. He also believed that doctors exposed to a patient with an infection should avoid contact with pregnant women for six months.

The medical community responded with derision. We probably shouldn't be surprised that doctors would resist embracing a theory that made them the culprits in the deaths of so many mothers and their children. A leading obstetrician, Dr. Charles Meigs, dismissed Holmes' work because, he wrote, doctors are gentlemen and "gentlemen's hands are clean."

Holmes' recommendations for preventing childbirth infections were better received in England than in America. Despite mockery from the medical establishment in his own country, he was heard and respected elsewhere. The same can't be said of our next hero.

Semmelweis—Savior of Mothers

A portrait of Ignaz Semmelweis hangs on the wall of the conference room of a hospital obstetrics department near my home in Florida. Today called the "savior of mothers," in the 1840s he was in charge of two birthing clinics attached to a hospital in Vienna. The clinics were teaching institutions that gave free healthcare to poor women and their babies. One clinic was staffed by men who were doctors and medical students, and the other by women who were midwives and their apprentices.

The two clinics used identical methods, yet the facility staffed by men had more than twice the rate of death from puerperal fever—a fact known to the public. The clinics admitted women for childbirth on alternate days, so women did their best to give birth on days when the midwives were accepting patients.

So great was the preference for the midwives' clinic that some women who expected to deliver on a day when only the doctors' clinic was open would let their babies be born at home. Then they would check into the midwives' clinic the next day and claim they had delivered while on the way to the hospital. The ruse qualified a baby to receive post-natal care from the midwives.

Semmelweis noticed something that added to the puzzle. The "in route" deliveries had lower rates of puerperal infection than births at *either* of the clinics. He started keeping records.

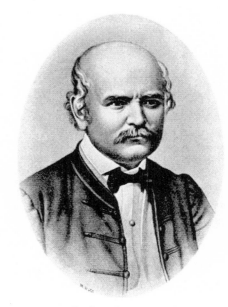

Dr. Ignaz Semmelweis
(Source: Encyclopedia Britannica)

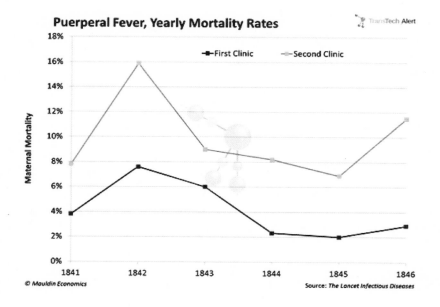

When a good friend died of puerperal fever after being cut by a scalpel used in the autopsy of a woman who had succumbed to that disease, Semmelweis concluded that some unknown contaminant, which he called cadaverous particles, was responsible for the two infections and for puerperal fever generally.

Differences in the practices of the two clinics provided another clue. The midwives' clinic performed no autopsies, so there was little opportunity for infection from corpses. Additionally, the midwives, who took no delight in displaying the gore of their profession, were much more likely to wash their hands and change aprons between deliveries.

Semmelweis instituted a rule requiring clinic workers to wash their hands with a solution of calcium hypochlorite. Though the chemical's antiseptic properties were entirely unknown, it was understood that the chemical destroyed the foul odors associated with the rotting flesh of cadavers.[15]

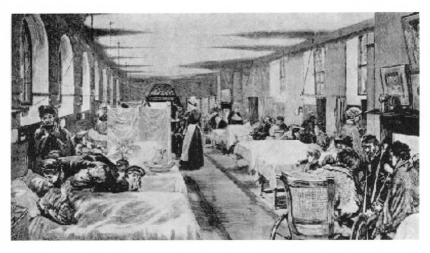

Typical clinic setting conducive to the spreading of childbed fever.
(Source: Indiana University)

As soon as the hand-washing rule was implemented, deaths from puerperal fever plummeted to less than one-tenth their previous level. In March and August of 1848, no woman died in childbirth in either of

15 Calcium hypochlorite is used to this day to treat swimming pool water; most readers would recognize its chlorine smell.
http://www.britannica.com/EBchecked/topic/534198/Ignaz-Philipp-Semmelweis

Semmelweis's clinics. This chart based on the historical data tells the story eloquently.

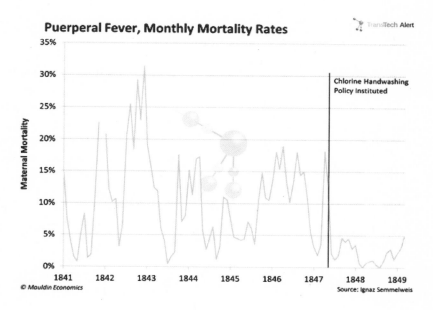

Puerperal Fever, Monthly Mortality Rates

TransTech Alert

Chlorine Handwashing Policy Instituted

© Mauldin Economics   Source: Ignaz Semmelweis

It's difficult to overstate the importance of this breakthrough, which could have saved millions of women's lives—if only it had been widely accepted. Semmelweis should have been celebrated as a hero when he published his data. The courts of Europe should have granted him titles and awards.

But that's not what happened. Today, hospitals are named after Ignaz Semmelweis, movies have told his story, and statues testify to his contribution to human health. At the time, however, he offended deeply held beliefs of the medical community, which was proud of its professional skepticism and reluctant to admit that anything as simple as hand washing could spare so many mothers from death.

Criticism of Semmelweis and his work was constant and cruel. Frustrated and obsessed with the refusal of the medical establishment to look at his evidence, in 1865 he s uffered a mental breakdown.[16] After a journey to Vienna urged by friends and relatives, he was committed to an

16 http://www.encyclopedia.com/topic/Ignaz_Philipp_Semmelweis.aspx

asylum. He died there just two weeks later, ironically from an infected cut on his finger that led to a generalized sepsis similar to that of puerperal fever.

Today the term "Semmelweis reflex" refers to bigoted opposition to any discovery that clashes too jarringly with what people believe.

Despite Semmelweis's own martyrdom, his work continued to attract attention and influence medical practices. Decades later, the ingenious Louis Pasteur proved that Semmelweis had been right by demonstrating the existence of disease-causing microorganisms.

Pasteur succeeded in being heard, but the way for that success had been prepared by others. Joseph Lister's antiseptic surgical techniques had drastically cut post-surgical infections and produced persuasive evidence for the germ theory. And the impact of Semmelweis's work—whereby many doctors began to adopt the practice of antiseptic hand washing, generally without acknowledging that Semmelweis had been right—had slowly accumulated.

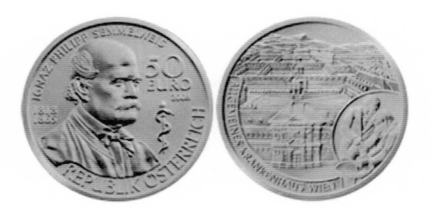

Regardless, the acceptance of the germ theory in the late 1800s truly revolutionized medicine. But it was only a matter of time until that immensely important new knowledge ossified into dogma that hindered further discovery.

Chapter 18

Joseph Goldberger and the Pellagra Plague

J oseph Goldberger and his parents came to America from Czechoslovakia when he was a boy. In 1892, he enrolled in what is now New York University School of Medicine. By that time, germ theory had already changed the practice of medicine and the study of epidemics.

Goldberger was drawn to epidemiology and eventually moved among research positions in Puerto Rico, Mexico, Mississippi and Louisiana. His work focused on the scourges of his era, including measles, yellow fever, typhus, and typhoid fever. His research on the transmission of disease by parasites is still studied.

Because Goldberger was so successful in studying and identifying the germs responsible for infectious diseases, the US Surgeon General recruited him in 1914 to confront an epidemic of pellagra in the American South.

Unless you work in the medical field, odds are you've never heard of this largely forgotten disease. Its name comes from the Italian "pelle" (skin) and "agra" (rough). It can be deadly: a medical school mnemonic for pellagra was the four Ds: dermatitis, diarrhea, dementia and death.[17] In the first half of the twentieth century, at least 100,000 Americans died of it.

In the early 1900s, pellagra was rampant in the South, where at least three million people were afflicted. At its peak, more than half of the inmates of mental institutions in the South had the disease. The condition also reached epidemic levels in much of rural Europe. Because diet in these areas centered on corn, it was suspected that the plant carried a pathogen responsible for the disease or that insects infesting corn were spreading a pathogen. Corn itself wasn't considered as a possible cause because among

---

17 Because the disfiguring disease was first described by 16th-century scientists in the Spanish province of Asturias, it was also called Asturian leprosy.

cultures relying even more heavily on the grain, Mesoamerican Indians from Mexico to Costa Rica, pellagra was unknown.

Goldberger, however, rejected germs as the cause of pellagra. He saw that it was a disease of the poor, such as children in orphanages, who were fed cheap foods. Though he lacked the opportunity for double-blind trials, he advanced his no-germ theory by inducing pellagra in a group of prisoners by limiting their diets to grits and a few other foods such as cabbage, sweet potatoes and rice.

In 1915, Goldberger published his initial results. They were ignored or rejected by those who insisted that disease comes from germs, so some germ must be responsible for pellagra.[18]

Goldberger's theory did have supporters, however. So dedicated were they to stopping the easily prevented illness that they held "pellagra parties." These grisly gatherings featured nutritional crusaders eating the scabs of pellagra victims to demonstrate their confidence that the condition was not a germ-driven, communicable disease.

Finally, in 1937, American biochemist Conrad Elvehjem produced pellagra in dogs by limiting them to a diet deficient in niacin, or vitamin B3. In corn, that vitamin is concentrated in the outer layers of the kernel, which in the US and Europe was routinely removed to retard the spoilage of cornmeal. The reason corn's role in the pellagra puzzle had been so confusing was that disease-free Mesoamericans cooked the grain in a way that conserved the niacin.[19]

Perhaps the richest form of easily available niacin is the yeast left over from brewing beer. When the importance of the B-complex vitamins became public knowledge, food manufacturers developed a variety of products to satisfy consumer demand, including Vegemite and Marmite, which remain popular in Australia today.

The vitamin B3 controversy is far from unique. Throughout modern history, nutritional discoveries have been made, mocked, embraced, and then forgotten. The long, bizarre story of vitamin C has inspired books, including one by a Nobel laureate. And a controversy about optimal levels of vitamin D is raging in scientific circles right now, where we see the same reticence among older scientists to admit they've hurt public health by shunning new evidence.

---

18 Historians of science speculate today that resistance to his research was due in part to the indifference of scientific and civil authorities to the plight of the largely black poor.
19 The process is known as nixtamalization, which involves soaking the corn in an alkaline solution.

Chapter 19

Shining Light on the
Sunshine Vitamin

The scientific consensus that has held sway for four decades about sun exposure and vitamin D has collapsed. What has emerged in place of the old, "settled science" is research showing that most people in North America are seriously deficient in vitamin D. The same is true for Northern Europe, and the implications are staggering.

Simply put, it means that unless you're one of the few people with optimal serum D levels—such as lifeguards and roofers in South Florida—you can cut your risk from most major diseases by 50 to 80 percent just by getting enough vitamin D. Moreover, people with darker skin manufacture less vitamin D, so they likely would gain even more from reaching optimum vitamin D levels.

The recent findings on vitamin D mean we can significantly reduce healthcare costs by taking a few simple steps. If researchers are right, the benefits of raising the level of vitamin D in your blood (serum D levels) from the less than 25 nanograms per milliliter typical of Americans to about 45 ng/ml are enormous. Even if they're wrong, risks from the recommended therapy are trivial to nonexistent.

If you research this subject for yourself, you will encounter holdouts who insist that exposure to sunlight is always dangerous and that a normal diet supplemented by a daily multivitamin provides enough vitamin D. Behind the scenes, however, even the National Institutes of Health (NIH) has shifted its position on vitamin D, but without taking too much blame for having resisted the evidence for decades.

Dr. Michael Holick, the researcher most responsible for the radical change in thinking, calls vitamin D deficiency a "silent epidemic." It goes unnoticed because there are no stark symptoms. Instead, vitamin D deficiency raises the incidence of virtually all diseases.

The substance has been a newsmaker for more than a century.

In the 1890s, a crippling, bone-softening children's disease called "rickets" was still widespread in the Northeastern states, a region with a thicker ozone layer than the Northwest. Ozone blocks the invisible component of sunshine, ultraviolet B (UVB), which is the light that prompts vitamin D production in the skin.

In the early 1900s, it was demonstrated that exposure to midday summer sunshine prevented rickets. There was an effort to educate the public about the discovery, and nearly everybody learned that a little sunshine was good for you. If you're of baby boomer age, your mother undoubtedly told you to go outside and get some sun. Now you know why.

Ironically, the beginning of the end of this attitude came in 1923, when Professor Harry Steenbock at University of Wisconsin-Madison discovered that ultraviolet (UV) irradiation could boost the vitamin D content of milk and other foods. The practice of enriching milk became routine, and rickets all but disappeared. Slowly, something else disappeared—the notion that sunlight is healthy.

For the most part, scientists lost interest in the biological function of sunlight for higher animals. Dr. Michael Holick was the notable exception. For the last thirty years, Holick has been gathering data and studying the role of sunlight and vitamin D.

A Hormone Called a Vitamin

While still a graduate student, Holick identified the predominant form of vitamin D circulating in human blood as 25-hydroxyvitamin D.[20] Next he discovered the mechanism by which the skin synthesizes vitamin D and demonstrated the effects of aging, obesity, latitude, seasonal change, sunscreen use, skin pigmentation, and clothing on the process.

Thanks to his work, we now know that D is not really a vitamin. It is a "prohormone," meaning it's a precursor of a steroid hormone produced from D in the liver, kidneys, and lungs. This active hormone regulates important biological functions. *Every single cell in the body has a D receptor—even*

---

20 He later identified the active form of vitamin D as 1,25-dihydroxyvitamin D.

stem cells.

When I asked Holick about the source of his long-ago epiphany, he said it was the simple fact that D is a critical nutrient without a natural food source. It is biologically so important that early humans needed the ability to manufacture D even during famines.

For that reason, Holick questioned the conventional zero-tolerance approach to sun exposure that dermatologists have advocated since the 1970s. A professor of dermatology himself, he lost his teaching position when he published his findings. When he wrote a book on the subject, his message was targeted with a well funded debunking campaign by the leading dermatological organization. Supposedly objective journals refused to publish his exhaustive research—research now accepted as accurate and pioneering.

Fortunately, the vitamin D climate has begun to change. Of late, Holick has received some of the recognition he deserves, and he now advises the National Institutes of Health (NIH). He also works as a professor of medicine, physiology and biophysics at Boston University School of Medicine.

Breakthroughs in other areas support Holick's case. With advances in computer processing and the decoding of the human genome, for example, *it now appears that the behaviors of 2,000 genes are influenced by vitamin D*.

The lessons of the rickets epidemic are only now sinking in. Mainstream medical thinking is finally beginning to recognize the connection between D and osteomalacia, which is essentially rickets of the aged. Dosages of D are being recommended at levels high enough to do for that disease what lower doses did for rickets. In fact, Dr. Holick and others have demonstrated that osteomalacia is preventable and treatable with vitamin D. Osteoporosisis also is related to vitamin D deficiency.

Bone disease is only a part of the story. Optimal vitamin D levels, whether attained through sunlight or supplementation, dramatically reduce the risk of breast cancer, colon cancer and melanoma skin cancer.

Yes, that's right. The incidence of these really nasty skin cancers can be reduced by moderate, sensible sunshine or vitamin D supplementation. Non-melanoma skin cancers do increase somewhat with sun exposure, especially with sunburn. Such skin cancers, however, are relatively unthreatening, as they tend not to spread to other parts of the body. Most are easily detected and removed because they appear on sun-exposed skin.

Melanoma, on the other hand, is deadly. We've been told that the risk increases with exposure to sunshine, yet melanoma frequently occurs on skin areas that get little direct sunlight. The bottom line, which is worth repeating, is that the incidence of melanoma goes down significantly with moderate exposure to UVB-containing sunshine or with vitamin D3 supplementation. Vitamin D also improves skin tone.

All the big killers and expensive diseases are ameliorated by adequate D, including hypertension, cardiovascular disease and stroke. So are type-1 (and, to a lesser extent, type-2) diabetes, rheumatoid arthritis, peripheral vascular disease, multiple sclerosis, dementia, autoimmune diseases, and apparently even viral diseases such as H1N1 flu and AIDS.

Most adults need to take in about 4,000 international units (IUs) of D per day. You'll need even more if you are obese, are taking certain medicines or have a condition that hampers production of usable D. According to the American Society for Clinical Nutrition, consuming up to 10,000 IU of vitamin D per day has no adverse effects except for individuals with certain identifiable conditions, such as hyperparathyroidism or abnormal calcium excretion.[21]

Adults who move from the level of deficiency that is now widespread to optimal vitamin D levels can increase their life expectancy by six to eight years—and cut their medical bills. The Canadians seem to be well ahead of Americans in terms of understanding the cost of vitamin D deficiency and have estimated potential healthcare savings in that country to be as high as $50 billion annually, or $1,400 per person per year.

A sound estimate of annual savings in direct and indirect health costs from widespread adoption of vitamin D therapy in the U.S. would be difficult to produce, due to the financial complexity of the U.S. medical system. Whatever the number, it would be a big one, perhaps 20% to 30% of total medical costs.

For a good but complex overview of the kinds of healthcare benefits from optimal vitamin D, I recommend this video by the Canadian scientist, William B. Grant, PhD. http://uctv.tv/shows/Cost-Benefit-of-Optimal-Health-with-Sunshine-Vitamin-D-29082

---

21 See http://ajcn.nutrition.org/content/69/5/842.full

All-Round Life Enhancer

The availability of natural UVB depends on the latitude where you live. Holick judges that from Los Angeles south, sunshine provides adequate UVB year round. But in more northerly latitudes, not even the palest among us will get sufficient UVB from sunshine, excepting, perhaps, farmers who till in the nude. In Boston or Montreal, for example, levels of UVB that people receive are negligible from mid-October through mid-April. Even young people can barely store enough D during summer months to make it through the winter. Older people can't get close.

For the deficient, the benefits of vitamin D therapy appear rapidly. Holick and others who prescribe D report that patients often experience dramatic health improvements within months. Not only do hypertension and bone density respond quickly, so do neuralgia and muscular weakness. Depression, irritable bowel syndrome and other maladies also may respond promptly to the sunshine vitamin.

Chapter 20

Coffee: The Revolutionary Beverage

N ot all scientific discoveries come from the lab. The biotech revolution is providing computational and analytical tools that enable scientists to locate solutions hiding in plain sight. None is more interesting than coffee.

Java Jive

I often hear people tell me they've given up coffee "for my health." Given my lack of tact and my general paucity of social skills, the announcement throws me into desperate inner conflict. Usually I'm able to curb my impulses and simply ask about the evidence that coffee is unhealthy. I've never gotten an answer that makes sense. Occasionally, someone will say he felt dependent on caffeine and took the dependency to be unhealthy, though we all depend on a variety of biological and nutritional components.

So let's pour a cup.

Some historians have proposed that the introduction of coffee to the West contributed both to the Enlightenment and to its offshoot, the American Revolution. The idea is not such a stretch.

In medieval Britain, drinking beer was a strategy for avoiding water-borne disease. Though alcohol at the usual concentrations in beer won't kill all pathogens, it does slow them down, and it keeps them from growing at all in beer that has been pasteurized.

When coffee came onto the British scene in the 1500s, it offered another way to take water safely. As with preparing tea, pathogens were killed by boiling the water.

In those days, coffee was much more expensive than tea, and few people had experience brewing the stuff, so coffeehouses sprang up. They generally didn't sell by the cup. Rather, they collected a cover charge, after which the java flowed freely. Hyperactive coffee drinkers began to pop up in place of quasi-sedated beer drinkers.

Students and merchants found these establishments pleasant spots to study, do business and talk. Since none of them had a Wi-Fi connection, merchants who tracked the world's happenings and their impact on business would announce news to the entire assemblage as they received it. Naturally, discussions turned to politics and philosophy. Arguments were advanced, and movements were born.

Edward Lloyd opened his Angel coffeehouse in 1650. The Oxford hangout of merchants and shippers evolved into insurance powerhouse Lloyd's of London. In Scotland, Enlightenment thinking flourished in coffeehouses where the sippers could share the works of Baruch Spinoza and Adam Smith.

Daniel Webster called the Boston coffeehouse, Green Dragon Tavern, "headquarters of the Revolution." Open from 1697 to 1832, it was frequented by John Adams, James Otis, and Paul Revere, who met there to conspire. The New York Stock Exchange and the Bank of New York began as coffeehouses.

Just as contemporary politicians would like to regulate political speech, especially on the Internet, the British Crown sought to dampen the exchange of free and often antiauthoritarian ideas that would wash through coffeehouses. In 1675, King Charles II issued "A proclamation for the suppression of coffee-houses."[22]

The justifications were helpfully included in the proclamation:

> Whereas it is most apparent, that the Multitude of Coffee-Houses of late years set up and kept within this Kingdom, the Dominion of Wales, and the Town of Berwick upon Tweed, and the great resort of idle and disaffected persons to them, have produced very evil and dangerous effects; as well for that many Tradesmen and others, do therein mis-spend much of their time, which might and probably would otherwise be imployed in and about their Lawful Callings and Affairs; but also, for that in such Houses, and by occasion of the meetings of such persons therein, diverse False, Malitious and Scandalous Reports are devised and spread abroad, to the Defamation of His Majesties Government, and to the Disturbance of the

---

22 http://www.staff.uni-giessen.de/gloning/tx/suppress.htm

Peace and Quiet of the Realm ..."

Coffee itself is still maligned today, though as a health problem. All over the world, there are efforts to stamp out the demon bean. But when I hear people say they've cut out coffee for the sake of their health, I'm baffled. The vague explanation given by most of the decaffeinated martyrs is that coffee must be bad for you. After all, it makes you alert and happy—two worrisome signs.

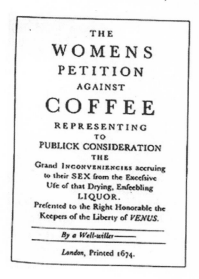

In truth, coffee is a health food. It is the primary source of antioxidants in the American diet, and I consider it the single most beneficial food item in most grocery stores.

I've spent a lot of time trying to understand how extreme opinions about diet and health gain such power with no actual evidence. It's nothing new, but now that we have instant access to peer-reviewed literature via Google Scholar[23], there's no excuse.

Anti-Alzheimer's Drink

I learned the most about coffee from Mark A. Smith, PhD, a professor of pathology at Case Western Reserve University.

Smith was no slouch. He served on the editorial boards of over 200 journals, including *Science Translational Medicine, Journal of Neurochemistry* and *American Journal of Pathology*. He was director of Basic Science Research at the University Memory and Aging Center and editor-in-chief of the *Journal of Alzheimer's Disease*. He was killed by a drunk driver in 2010, but his influence survives.

We weren't close friends, but he was always available with answers and was ready to talk about anything he considered important. One of those

23 https://scholar.google.co.uk/schhp

topics was the efficacy of coffee as a disease preventative and life extender.

Scientists of his standing have a reputation for reluctance to speak plainly, but Smith was surprisingly frank in his endorsement of coffee. Even better, as editor-in-chief of the *Journal of Alzheimer's Disease*, he published a special issue on "Therapeutic Opportunities for Caffeine in Alzheimer's Disease and Other Neurodegenerative Disorders."

The *JAD* is an authoritative and pricey publication. But Dr. Smith so wanted to share what he had learned about by the power of coffee and caffeine that he distributed the issue for free. You can read it at http://content.iospress.com/journals/journal-of-alzheimers-disease/20/S1

At the very least, you should read these excerpts.

> Although caffeine is the most widely consumed psychoactive drug worldwide, its potential beneficial effect for maintenance of proper brain functioning has only recently begun to be adequately appreciated. This has mainly resulted from the convergence of conclusions from epidemiological studies and from fundamental research in animal models. Epidemiological studies first revealed an inverse association between the chronic consumption of caffeine and the incidence of Parkinson's disease; this was paralleled by animal studies of Parkinson's disease showing that caffeine prevented motor deficits as well as neurodegeneration. Later a few epidemiological studies showed that *the consumption of moderate amounts of caffeine was inversely associated with the cognitive decline associated with aging as well as the incidence of Alzheimer's disease*. Again, this was paralleled by animal studies showing that chronic caffeine administration prevented memory deterioration and neurodegeneration in animal models of aging and of Alzheimer's disease. [Emphasis mine]

Also...

> Caffeine seems particularly effective to normalize rather than bolstering memory performance and is a candidate disease-modifying agent for Alzheimer's disease, based on its neuroprotective profile and its ability to reduce amyloid-beta production. Although an inverse relationship between caffeine consumption and neurodegenerative disorders appeared compelling, it was consensual that several methodological issues must be solved before advancing to decisive clinical trials.

Because caffeine is a naturally occurring substance and therefore can't be patented, it's unlikely anyone will invest the many millions of dollars needed to obtain FDA approval to sell it as a drug. Moreover, others have shown that bare caffeine doesn't deliver the benefits to be gained from the full molecular cocktail we call coffee.

The abstract for the chapter titled "Caffeine and Coffee as Therapeutics Against Alzheimer's Disease"[24] contains these remarkable words:

> Caffeine appears to provide its disease-modifying effects through multiple mechanisms, including a direct reduction of A-beta production through suppression of both beta- and gamma-secretase levels. These results indicate a surprising ability of moderate caffeine intake (the human equivalent of 500 mg caffeine or 5 cups of coffee per day) to protect against or treat AD in a mouse model for the disease and a therapeutic potential for caffeine against AD in humans.

Notice the term "disease-modifying." It means that the mechanisms of Alzheimer's are reversed. There is a $6 billion market today for Alzheimer's drugs that are not disease-modifying.

There's more. The issue's chapter on "Caffeine, Diabetes, Cognition, and Dementia"[25] surveys the evidence that coffee protects against type-2 diabetes. In fact, coffee may protect against other maladies as well, including liver and heart diseases, though they are not the focus of this particular article.

The *JAD* issue emphasized the need for further research to discover how coffee and caffeine work, and since then, there's been really interesting progress.

Coffee Activates the Guardian Angel Gene

A healthy body sweeps away its own mess. The boost that coffee can give to the process is explained by a February 2011 article in the journal *Autophagy* titled "Caffeine Induces Apoptosis by Enhancement of Autophagy via PI3K/Akt/mTOR/p70S6K Inhibition."[26] It's not an easy read, though, so let me give you a quick summary.

The authors document the role of caffeine in autophagy or "self-eating."

---

24 http://www.ncbi.nlm.nih.gov/pubmed/20182037
25 http://www.ncbi.nlm.nih.gov/pubmed/20182038
26 http://www.ncbi.nlm.nih.gov/pmc/articles/PMC3039768/

Sounds gruesome, but autophagy is a cell function that protects the health of the organism of which the cell is a part. When an element of a cell is worn out or has become irreparably flawed from age or injury, the best service the cell can give the organism is to shut down and, if possible, give up its components for recycling.

Autophagy follows *apoptosis*, or cell suicide. It may seem counterintuitive, but cell suicide is our friend. A mutated cell that fails to commit apoptosis and die might go on replicating and become a cancer.

Apoptosis is a function of the "guardian angel gene," p53, which serves as the master regulator of genomic repair or suicide. All cancers rely on blocking the operation of the p53 gene. Caffeine is an activator of p53, which may explain some of the health benefits associated with coffee and tea.

As the abstract for this paper in the *Journal of Cancer Research*[27] states, "The same low concentration of caffeine that was effective for inducing phosphorylation of p53 was also shown to increase p53 activation."

Autophagy is also triggered by calorie restriction, which is the best-proven life extension strategy so far. Even in primate studies, calorie restriction with optimal nutrition (CRON) improves health. Of course, CRON also leaves people chronically hungry, so there will probably never be a long-term human study. A very few people manage to cut calorie intake to the bare minimum for years at a time, but only a very few. That's why it's such great news that caffeine may be a p53 activator, even if you eat donuts by the dozen.

Not Just Coffee

Caffeine is not the only way to induce the effects of CRON without going hungry. Several mitochondrial enhancers seem to replicate "winter," or calorie-restricted states, in animals. Nicotinamide riboside (NR), which I've already mentioned, and oxaloacetate both increase mitochondrial function and activate some of the genes that are turned on via calorie restriction. Both compounds are manufactured naturally in our cells and in the last few years have been synthesized as dietary supplements.

---

27 cancerres.aacrjournals.org/content/63/15/4396.short

The data is strong enough that I've begun taking NR and oxaloacetate as dietary supplements myself. However, evidence is mounting that the easiest and most pleasurable way to take a mitochondrial-enhancing compound is much simpler—your morning coffee.

One last thing: Some people can easily drink a lot of coffee and some cannot. I've had my genome analyzed by some of the best scientists, so I know I have none of the alleles known to cause adverse reactions to caffeine. This may not be true for you. My wife can only drink modest amounts of coffee without hurting her sleep.

Getting in Touch with Your Genome

I'd like to tell you to talk to your geneticist about the benefits of drinking coffee, but that probably won't be practical for a year or two, until a company I've written about in my newsletter, *Transformational Technology Alert*, is ready for large-scale operations. In the meantime, use your own discretion. And talk to your doctor about coffee. If nothing else, you'll find out whether he's keeping up with the literature.

By the way, blueberries contain a natural anti-fungal called pterostilbene that seems to be extremely effective as a CRON pathway activator. A cocrystallized compound combining pterostilbine and caffeine called PURENERGY stays active in the system longer than simple caffeine and also makes caffeine easier to take for those subject to "the jitters."

The tenacious ignorance about coffee is a limp reenactment of the treatment of Ignaz Semmelweis. You may not think that we, in our modern era, would punish scientists as Semmelweis was punished. However, the government would treat any coffee company that dared to repeat the *JAD's* statements about the disease-modifying impacts of the bean as a criminal organization. Multiple federal agencies would descend, beat the company to death, and lock up its management in the Semmelweis Correctional Facility.

Chapter 21

Caution That Kills

We accept our modern institutions, policies, and attitudes as being more or less what they should be, just as the people of 17th-century Vienna did theirs. Austrians of the 1800s believed they were living in thoroughly modern times, so evidence that failing to wash one's hands with chlorine bleach might be a colossal, death-dealing mistake was dismissed.

Today hundreds of millions of people live in poor health or die early because institutions, often governmental, suppress simple facts about nutrition and resist the development and use of new therapies. What keeps this large-scale tragedy rolling on, year after year, is the desire to avoid embarrassing established "experts," inconveniencing political or business allies or taking on the thankless t,ask of exposing popular beliefs as mere superstition and psychological inertia.

The excuse you'll get from all the willing participants is that it's better to err on the side of caution, and much of the public buys that alibi. They've heard the Hippocratic maxim, "First do no harm," and they accept it as a reason for a hyper-cautious appraisal of any new therapy.

They are wrong. They are joining in a mistake that in the 21st century leads to deaths that are as avoidable as the deaths of mothers in the filthy birthing clinics of the 18th century.

I hope you don't misunderstand me; gullibility is no virtue. Nor, however, is unbending skepticism a virtue. On the contrary, such skepticism is the enemy of an open mind. It resists and wants to suppress anything that is more than slightly new.

Isaac Asimov, whom I was privileged to know years ago, held a remarkable view of scientific history. Though best known for his science fiction stories, he wrote much else. He was primarily a science writer, perhaps the greatest in history, with about 500 nonfiction books.

He famously said, "Your assumptions are your windows on the world. Scrub them off every once in a while, or the light won't come in."

That is not an invitation to abandon critical, scientific thought. Rather, it invites a skeptical but open mind to benefit from rapidly developing science and technology.

Skeptics and the Shortness of Life

Don't take my word for it, though. Instead, I urge you to consider the counsel of "the father of empiricism," the scientist whose demand for evidenced-based thinking set the stage for the scientific method, the Enlightenment, and eventually the modern technologies we benefit from today: Francis Bacon.

Bacon didn't advise stubborn resistance to new ideas or pride in such an attitude. In the *Novum Organum Scientiarum* (The New Instrument of Science), he wrote:

> But by far the greatest obstacle to the progress of science and to the undertaking of new tasks and provinces therein is found in this—that men despair and think things impossible. For wise and serious men are wont in these matters to be altogether distrustful, considering with themselves the obscurity of nature, the shortness of life, the deceitfulness of the senses, the weakness of the judgment, the difficulty of experiment, and the like; and so supposing that in the revolution of time and of the ages of the world the sciences have their ebbs and flows; that at one season they grow and flourish, at another wither and decay, yet in such sort that when they have reached a certain point and condition they can advance no further. If therefore anyone believes or promises more, they think this comes of an ungoverned and unripened mind, and that such attempts have prosperous beginnings, become difficult as they go on, and end in confusion.

Bacon understood how "the shortness of life" contributes to unreasoning skepticism. Even intelligent and generally positive people tend to get discouraged and depressed as the shadow of their own mortality advances.

In the terminology of psychoanalysis, this is *projection*. We tend to project our own fears and failures onto the larger world. In every generation, we see older people turn bitter and pessimistic, predicting the demise of civilization along with themselves.

That doesn't happen to everyone, though. Many great thinkers maintain a youthful confidence in humanity's abilities, even as they succumb to the last challenges of illness and death. Ironically, we live in a time when an increasing number of scientists view even those challenges as addressable.

As I've already pointed out, health spans have grown exponentially for several centuries. If, as I believe, we are heading toward the near-vertical portion of the exponential curve, it is within reach for even the elderly to extend their productive health spans. This makes the process of discovery rather urgent, at least for those of us who are old. In the next part of the book, I'll explain some of the remarkable breakthroughs that have already occurred.

These transformational biotechnologies *will* make it to market.

The recent deregulation of stem cell medicine in Japan is just the start. Some international players are already preparing to make innovative therapies available to those who need them most urgently. Health tourism is globalizing biotech and subverting institutional resistance to change. Revolutionary life-extending biotechnologies don't have to wait on reforms in the US.

For most people, the greatest challenge to benefiting from new science is internal: overcoming the mob instinct that rejects and attacks anything that is truly radical. Here's a quote from someone with more credibility than I'll ever have, the ingenious Louis Pasteur.

> Young men, have confidence in those powerful and safe methods, of which we do not yet know all the secrets. And, whatever your career may be, do not let yourselves become tainted by a deprecating and barren scepticism, do not let yourselves be discouraged by the sadness of certain hours which pass over nations.
> —The life of Pasteur (1911), Volume II. p. 228

PART III:

The Biotech Singularity

Chapter 22

One Less Worry

As you've seen in Part I, big changes are on the way—bigger than most people can imagine. Science is progressing at an unprecedented rate. The old, recalcitrant habits of thought and regulation eventually will be swept aside, and the imperative to hold on to life will prevail. Nothing can stop the transformation of medicine, not even the errors of great minds.

In 2005, futurist Ray Kurzweil published *The Singularity Is Near—When Humans Transcend Biology*. He predicted an acceleration in technological progress that by 2045 would outrace mankind's ability to comprehend it. For many, however, "the singularity" has been narrowed to mean the emergence of super-intelligent machines able to dominate humans and seize control of our fate.

Movies like the *Terminator* series and *The Matrix* trilogy play into the fear of artificial intelligence, or AI. Some who are fanning the fear of self-conscious computers are extremely influential. I wish they'd focus instead on the very real challenges presented by the flipping of the demographic pyramid.

It's easier to fuss over imaginary threats than to deal with real problems. For most of my life, people in society's highest circles were convinced that overpopulation was humanity's biggest problem—despite clear evidence that the world was moving toward depopulation. Only in recent years did headlines report "Germany Fights Population Drop," or "Sex Education in Europe Turns to Urging More Births," or "Italy Is a 'Dying Country' Says Minister as Birth Rate Plummets."

And not that long ago, investors lost money because they believed the widely disseminated nonsense of "peak oil." Most of the establishment's dicta about diet and nutrition have been wrong if not actually harmful. Climate "science" has been taken over by fact-dodging politicians. The current fretting over a hypothetical threat from sentient machines, especially by the superstars of Silicon Valley, is just one more entry in the list of follies—a sad misallocation of intellectual and financial resources that could better be used to develop AI's potential for extending healthy lives.

"AIs," which are pieces of software found in everything from computer games to search engines, are not the self-aware and potentially malevolent "Sentient AI" computer systems of science-fiction. They won't bite you.

Turing Test

It all started with Alan Turing, the British genius, mathematician and cryptanalyst who, according to Winston Churchill, contributed more to Allied victory in World War II than any other individual. During that war, he designed pioneering computers capable of decrypting coded Nazi messages. *The Imitation Game* is only the most recent movie about Turing's remarkable and tragic life.

Turing was fascinated with artificial intelligence and in a 1950 paper, *Computing Machinery and Intelligence*[28], explained a game to help detect whether a computer is actually thinking. He proposed that if a computer, communicating via written messages, could convince more than 30% of a panel of judges that the messages were coming from a human, it might be "thinking."

In June 2014, a Russian supercomputer convinced judges at the Royal Society in London that they were chatting with a 13-year-old boy. Thus the machine passed the Turing Test.

Turing's name alone lends weight to claims that a computer has achieved the ability to think. After all, Turing, along with Hungarian-American scientist John von Neumann, originated the concepts underlying modern computers. So media reaction to the Russian computer's success was immediate and forceful. Initial coverage implied that the arrival of science-fiction-like AIs—silicon people—was imminent. Some stories raised the specter of Skynet, the evil machine intelligence of James Cameron's *Terminator* series that was bent on eradicating humankind.

After a few days, however, skeptical voices emerged about "Eugene

---

28 http://loebner.net/Prizef/TuringArticle.html

Goostman," the chat bot that helped trick a third of the judges in the Turing Test. I say it "helped trick" because the bot's designers gamed the test by telling the judges they'd be talking to a 13-year-old Ukrainian boy who could barely speak English. This fiction lowered the judges' expectations about the bot's language skills and cultural knowledge and provided perfect cover for non-sequiturs and misunderstandings that otherwise would have tipped them off to the nature of the chat. The disinformation worked.

While some in the media began to doubt the validity of the Eugene Goostman experiment, the goal of the test itself—to detect computers with true human abilities—was never questioned. Even now, most discussion about the Turing Test assumes that Sentient AIs will emerge at some point and that conscious computers may be just around the corner.

These predictions are encouraged by Moore's Law, which implies that the cost of packing more and more transistors into a computer will continue to plummet. The assumption is that a computer, having as many transistors as the brain has biological switches will be able to learn the way humans learn and will achieve self-awareness.

I don't believe it. In my opinion, the notion of a parallel between transistors and neurons shows that computer scientists completely misunderstand and underestimate the human mind.

To be fair, I'm not pinning that mistake on Alan Turing, although some of the predictions in his original paper have turned out to be wrong. The following excerpt includes such a critical failed prediction and illustrates the flaw behind the idea that thinking machines are possible if not inevitable.

> It will simplify matters for the reader if I explain first my own beliefs... Consider first the more accurate form of the question. I believe that in about fifty years' time it will be possible, to programme computers, with a storage capacity of about 10^9, to make them play the imitation game so well that an average interrogator will not have more than 70 per cent chance of making the right identification after five minutes of questioning. The original question, 'Can machines think?' I believe to be too meaningless to deserve discussion. Nevertheless I believe that at the end of the century the use of words and general educated opinion will have altered so much that one will be able to speak of machines thinking without expecting to be contradicted.

Clearly, he was off. There was no "general educated opinion" about thinking machines at the end of the century, nor is there now. While machines today can calculate extraordinarily well, nobody I know in computer science believes that computers do anything but follow instructions very quickly—adding machines operating at electronic speeds. It's possible to write software that allows a computer to "learn" new functions, but that's not thinking.

So why do so many people await the emergence of sentient super-machines?

Hacking Skynet

You can glean a lot about Turing's key misunderstanding from his thoughts about how to develop a program capable of passing the test that bears his name. What he proposed was not that programmers create a computer (software, actually) that can have an adult conversation. Rather, he envisioned computers and software capable of learning just as human babies do.

> Instead of trying to produce a programme to simulate the adult mind, why not rather try to produce one which simulates the child's? If this were then subjected to an appropriate course of education one would obtain the adult brain. Presumably the child brain is something like a notebook as one buys it from the stationer's. Rather little mechanism, and lots of blank sheets. (Mechanism and writing are from our point of view almost synonymous.) Our hope is that there is so little mechanism in the child brain that something like it can be easily programmed. The amount of work in the education we can assume, as a first approximation, to be much the same as for the human child.

Turing assumed that the only real requirement for thinking machines was the development of more sophisticated hardware. Where he and others after him went wrong was in failing to appreciate the unimaginable complexity of the human brain.

I feel, by the way, an urge to defend Turing. His misconceptions about a child's mind can be explained and excused by the primitive state of biological knowledge at the time he was writing. His thesis that the child's brain is so undeveloped "that something like it can be easily programmed" is so wrong, it strikes me as slightly humorous. Numerous smart and well-funded computer scientists have tried to create computers that could, like children, absorb educational input and develop a unified world view that could be communicated via language. None has come close.

In fact, humans emerge from the womb with an astonishingly developed "mechanism." On the surface, we see instincts like the fear of falling and the desire for nurturing. Beneath the surface, there is far more—including complex social skills and the basis of grammar. Children who aren't taught language will effortlessly develop their own ideoglossias[29] complete with sophisticated grammatical structures.

In his book, *The Language Instinct: How the Mind Creates Language*, cognitive scientist Steven Pinker points out that all of mankind, even isolated tribes, share the same basic rules of grammar. There has never been a human community, not even a small, isolated tribe, without highly complex language. We were equipped for complex language at birth.

The "mechanism" or genomic operating system goes far beyond language, though. We tend to take our many human instincts for granted because they're the water we swim in, but they're powerful. I'll give you a simple example.

When my daughter was born, I found that the scientific literature about the differences between boys and girls was true. Girls tend to have better fine motor control and physical skill, at least initially. I was amazed that within days of her birth, my daughter was able to focus her eyes and recognize the faces of family members. My son took weeks to reach that point, but my daughter was looking straight into our eyes the day we brought her home from the hospital. She also gave us fully developed recognition smiles that accomplished exactly what they were designed to do: complete ownership of her parents.

That's an example of "mechanism" that Turing overlooked. Strangers, by the way, caused my daughter noticeable anxiety. She turned away from people she didn't know, refusing to meet their eyes.

Once, when she was only a few weeks old, I held her on my lap in front of the TV. As the Spanish-language announcer introduced a musical act, the live audience cheered and clapped. My daughter had never heard or seen applause. Nevertheless, as soon as the TV crowd began to applaud, she tried to clap along with them. I still wonder about this fully developed and rather mysterious clapping instinct, clearly encoded in her DNA.

---

29 https://en.wikipedia.org/wiki/Idioglossia

When Turing wrote his paper, little was known about genetics. It was before 1953, and James Watson and Francis Crick hadn't yet discovered the double-helix of the DNA molecule. More importantly, we are only now beginning to understand the complexity of DNA information storage and processing.

The human genome consists of more than 3 billion base pairs of nucleotides, the letters the DNA code is written in. Included in that DNA are the 25,000 or so genes that are templates for assembling specific proteins. But those genes make up only a small part, about 1.5%, of the entire genome.

Not long ago, geneticists referred to the other 98.5% of the genome (that doesn't encode for proteins) as "junk." Today, however, they've identified four million gene switches in that junk that interact in ways that increase complexity to nearly incomprehensible levels. Somewhere in that impossibly complex code are mechanisms for language, music, smiling, and innumerable other capabilities that are ready to rip the moment the baby hits the air.

Bottom line: The task of building a computer equivalent of a human brain is vastly more difficult than programmers imagine. Perhaps it'll be possible—at some point in the future—for a machine to simulate the complexity of brain function delivered by the human genome. But I have my doubts.

Sentient AI: Not as Close as You Think

The brain can do what a system of on/off switches can do, so it's inviting to think of the brain as a computer. But we don't know where exactly those switches are or how they work and interact with one another.

As we unravel how the brain works on a cellular level, these biological systems prove to be more and more complex, so I don't believe we are anywhere near sentient artificial intelligence.

In fact, I'm not sure we will ever be able to create a real "artificial intelligence," with self-awareness and consciousness, out of silicon. It's impossible to say where intelligence starts and stops even in biological systems. We know a plant lacks intelligence, but animals are another matter. They're born with the instincts needed to survive in unforgiving environments. Perhaps a better test of machine consciousness would be whether a machine can duplicate animal survival and procreation in the wild—call it the Jungle Test.

The Eugene Goostman program does represent a step in a useful direction—not toward sentience but toward a better user interface, or UI. The backstop reason we don't have to fear Skynet is that UIs will trump AIs no matter how powerful AIs become.

Chapter 23

UI and AI Combined:
the Technology of the Future

D on't confuse advances in hardware with advances in the user interface. Yes, computers are smaller and faster now, but their basic functionality is little changed from a 1990 PC. The real change has been the in the ease of communicating with computers.

The Eugene Goostman exercise occurred almost exactly twenty years after Microsoft dropped support for DOS, the command-line user interface that preceded today's point-and-click interface. Personally, I miss DOS. For those who are willing to put in the work to learn complex instruction sets, command-line UIs are enormously powerful and fast. Few people care to, though, so easier ways of interacting with computers were developed. The mouse was the first great breakthrough. Today, especially in mobile computing, touch screens are an alternative to the mouse.

Programmers have put tremendous effort into developing an oral-language interface, and there has been progress. A family member who is a quadriplegic uses voice recognition software exclusively, mostly Dragon, even though the software doesn't yet work smoothly.

Google Voice is an AI that uses spoken language. In many ways, it's superior to the Eugene Goostman program because it doesn't waste resources trying to convince users it's something it's not. Like Siri, it works by going step by step through a complex logic tree similar to the flow charts students use in basic programming classes. This obviously is not thinking, although it does produce answers and so gives the appearance of thinking.

Here's an example of a simple flow-chart logic tree, provided by Wikipedia.

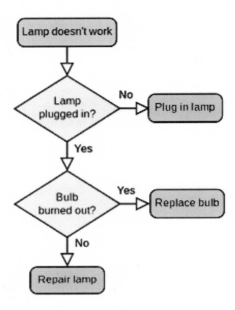

While this is a very simple tree, the elements have been applied to serious, complex problems. When there's a reason to go to the trouble and cost, a flow chart in software form can be sketched for almost any task.

Flow-chart logic is the basis of expert systems. The computer asks a series of questions about the situation and responds to the answers by following a logic tree that attempts to apply the decision-making process of an expert. As the answers accumulate, the expert system moves toward a solution. Such systems are extraordinarily useful, but they don't think. Nor will they in the foreseeable future.

AI Fearmongers

Like many others who fear a Sentient AI apocalypse, the brilliant entrepreneur Elon Musk cites the Swedish philosopher and economist Nick Bostrom. Bostrom is founding director of The Future of Humanity Institute and the Oxford Martin Programme on the Impacts of Future Technology at Oxford University.

To make sure you're getting both sides of the issue, I recommend this rather lengthy video of Bostrom's presentation at Google.[30] In it, he makes a lot of interesting points, but in the end gets several things very and verifiably wrong.

First, Bostrom dismisses life extension technologies as pure science-fiction, which demonstrates that news of recent developments in the biological sciences has not yet reached him. In fact, few of his fellow futurists have even a basic understanding of biology or genomics—a science that is changing everything we thought we knew about our brains and their true potential. (By the way, I've never encountered a biologist who believes machines are capable of true intelligence.)

Second, though Bostrom does acknowledge that it may be possible to merge biological and artificial intelligence, he brushes off the notion. But this emerging symbiosis between human and computer intelligence is, ultimately, the reason I'm not worried about Sentient AIs, malevolent or otherwise. We are rapidly approaching the time when keyboard, mouse, touchscreen, and voice recognition will all be replaced with direct brain interface (DBI). A human brain linked directly to a computer would trounce any AI system.

DBI: Direct Link to Unlimited Power?

The partnership between advanced computer technology and the human brain will always trump computer technology alone. Simply put, DNA + IA > IA. While this inequality is presented with tongue firmly in cheek, I'm quite serious about it.

Bostrom mentions direct brain interface technology, but again is dismissive of its progress and potential. Essentially, he says that he doesn't need a chip in his brain to Google something. He's missing the point. By harnessing pattern recognition, which is the human brain's greatest strength, DBIs will boost cognition, memory and processing power—and who knows what else.

What makes DBI so intriguing is that it recruits the power of the human brain.

---

30 https://youtu.be/pywF6ZzsghI

Already, retinal implants can feed information directly to the brain. With an existing commercial product, a chip implanted in the eye can receive visual data from a camera or even from a TV cable. Behind-the-scene, unpublished experiments have used implanted electrodes to transmit information directly to the vision center of the brain.

The development of virtual electrodes (through the manipulation of electrical fields between physical electrodes) to multiply the points of stimulation and enhance the rate of information flow is a particularly important area of DBI research. Such virtual electrodes are already being used in cochlear implants for the deaf.

That means we're not far from giving a human brain a seamless, bidirectional connection to a supercomputer. The biological resource this progress is tapping is the remarkable plasticity of the human brain. Results have surprised even the most optimistic researchers. It boils down to this: ***Human consciousness is so powerful and adaptable that it will take over any information processing system it is given access to.***

Even rat brains have shown a remarkable ability to co-opt computer systems, as have monkey brains. When scientists implant compasses or infrared vision in animal brains, the animals quickly learn to use them. This was all foretold, incidentally, by the experiences of people who suffered massive brain damage and then adapted other parts of the brain to restore lost functions.

Skynet, if it ever did emerge, would be hacked within minutes and be put to work relaying spam for an Eastern European or Chinese cybergang.

We all know that people are capable of enormous evil, as headlines demonstrate daily. I don't think sentient computers would present any more of a danger than evil people controlling increasingly powerful computers via DBI, who'd merge their malevolent human consciousness with machine capabilities. In fact, I don't see a big difference between the Skynet scenario and the direct control of supercomputers by the wrong humans.

Perhaps those on the right side of the ethical line should be encouraging research into the positive uses of the human/AI convergence as well as defenses against those who would misuse the technology.

Chapter 24

The Biotech Singularity

In the 1950s, John von Neumann, another pioneer of computer technology, anticipated Ray Kurzweil's concept of a technological singularity by half a century.

Born in Hungary in 1903, von Neumann moved in circles that included Albert Einstein, Richard Feynman, Edward Teller, James Watson, Francis Crick, Enrico Fermi, Niels Bohr, Robert Oppenheimer, and Max Planck. He played a key role in developing nuclear physics and was a pioneer in numerous fields—mathematics through functional analysis, economics through game theory and the minimax theorem, computing via von Neumann architecture, linear programming, stochastic computing and statistics.

Mathematician Stanislaw Ulam reported that a conversation with von Neumann "centered on the ever accelerating progress of technology and changes in the mode of human life, which give the appearance of approaching some essential singularity in the history of the race beyond which human affairs, as we know them, could not continue."

The key word here, I think, is "progress." By any measure, life in the modern era has improved remarkably. We live much longer, healthier lives. True want has been banished in the West and is rapidly disappearing in most of the rest of the world as well, as the following chart illustrates.

Today life is better for most Americans than it was for the wealthiest people only a generation ago. We have the whole of mankind's knowledge at our fingertips, and a worldwide communication network is wired up and waiting for anyone who wants to link in. Day-to-day tasks such as driving a car are much safer and cheaper. Food is so affordable that obesity has replaced malnutrition as the affliction of the poor. And already our institutions are overwhelmed by the growing costs of Social Security, Medicare and other transfer payments because people are living so long.

This progress will accelerate, and it is impossible to predict how it will change individual lives, institutions, nations, and the world. We're entering new territory, and no one can tell us what we'll find.

To understand why this is happening, listen to another of the great 20th-century scientists, Freeman Dyson.

Freeman Dyson: "Biology Is Now Bigger Than Physics"

Now in his nineties, Freeman Dyson is the sole survivor of the band of geniuses who transformed the last century. He knew and worked with virtually all the legends, including Albert Einstein and Richard Feynman. His best-known contributions to modern science were in mathematics, theoretical physics, quantum electrodynamics, solid-state physics, astronomy and nuclear engineering. He knows where progress in the 21st century is coming from.

In a 2007 essay[31] for *The New York Review of Books*, Dyson begins:

> It has become part of the accepted wisdom to say that the twentieth century was the century of physics and the twenty-first century will be the century of biology. Two facts about the coming century are agreed on by almost everyone. Biology is now bigger than physics, as measured by the size of budgets, by the size of the workforce, or by the output of major discoveries; and biology is likely to remain the biggest part of science through the twenty-first century. Biology is also more important than physics, as measured by its economic consequences, by its ethical implications, or by its effects on human welfare.

It would be hard if not impossible to better summarize the importance of modern biology.

Dyson has observed that the big physics problems had to be solved before biotechnology could be tackled successfully. Genomics and bioinformatics both depend on breakthroughs in physics that also support computer technology. Dyson himself speaks somewhat wistfully that he was kept from following his real biotech interests by physics problems that were more pressing.

---

31 http://www.nybooks.com/articles/2007/07/19/our-biotech-future/

Dyson expects that genetic engineering will supersede conventional manufacturing. Since chairs are made of an organic substance (wood), it should be possible to engineer plant DNA to grow wooden chairs. A farmer could grow a wooden plow from a seed.

I believe the potential is far greater than that—we could grow large structures such as houses and bridges, and they'd be self-repairing. According to Dyson, genetic engineering of this kind could decentralize manufacturing, to the benefit of places that are now sparsely populated but have plenty of sunlight.

Miniaturization of Biotech

Another Dyson idea that investors should note is the miniaturization of biotechnology, a process that will echo the transformation of the computer from a building-sized machine to a powerhouse that fits in a pocket.

When computers were big and expensive, IBM held a near monopoly. But it didn't bother to protect that position with patents, because it doubted that the market for computers would ever get big enough to attract competitors.

But then the miniaturization of components changed everything. It enabled Steve Wozniak and Steve Jobs to bring computing to the masses. Currently, the same process is taking place in biotech. Glow-in-the-dark plants that were genetically engineered by hobbyists are now being sold for profit, and far more consequential organisms are being developed.

I mentioned earlier that Novartis is investigating rapamycin's potential as an anti-aging drug. Rapamycin is produced by bacteria, and it's quite possible that researchers will discover other bacteria that produce molecules with life-extending properties. Or someone could design a bacterium to make an anti-aging molecule similar to rapamycin.

A decade ago, this could have been done only in the lab of a major company or university. Today, geeks are engineering bacteria at home with low-budget biotech tools. A recent *Popular Science* article on the DIY biohacker movement is titled "SXSW 2015: I Reprogrammed a Lifeform in Someone's Kitchen While Drinking a Beer." If this seems insignificant to you, I'm guessing you weren't an early investor in Apple.

One of the most important anti-aging compounds, anatabine citrate, was

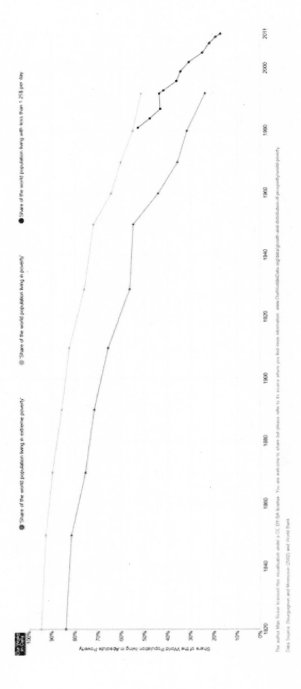

discovered by an amateur scientist without a college degree. Though the "inventor" was exceptional in having the resources to rent sophisticated biotech tools, the cost of such access has been plummeting for anyone who wants it.

In a few years, millions of people will have the tools to carry out sophisticated biological studies, just as millions of people today have the tools to write and test computer programs. The next wave of billionaire entrepreneurs, following in the footsteps of Jobs and Wozniak, will code with nucleotides (guanine, adenine, thymine, and cytosine) instead of with 0s and 1s.

Not all the big breakthroughs are in the future. In fact, some transformational technologies are in advanced stages of regulatory approval right now. By themselves they are enough to power progress of the sort John von Neumann was talking about when he said that human affairs as we know them could not continue.

So let's talk about some of what's making predicting the future so dicey.

Chapter 25

Cool Science

Scientists are making stunning progress toward understanding the cellular mechanisms of most major diseases. From cancer and liver disease to arthritis and Alzheimer's, recent discoveries will yield treatments that radically reduce the incidence and severity of disease.

One bright example of the wonderfully unexpected, remarkable advances being made is a "mechanical steroid." It's a machine that increases strength and endurance more effectively than the banned chemicals used by some elite athletes—and with none of the unhealthy side effects. It works by quickly drawing off the heat generated by muscle contraction, which greatly increases your capacity for exercise.

I've used the device, which is about the size of a coffee maker, for several years. Like many other early users, I've enjoyed remarkable improvement in strength, endurance and muscle mass. In fact, I'm physically more vigorous now than I was in my thirties, though the next-generation supplements that I've been taking probably play a role.

Not surprisingly, this biotechnology is spreading rapidly among professional athletes. The San Francisco 49ers and the Seattle Seahawks use it, as do the German national soccer team and some US Olympic training facilities. It also has been adopted as a training tool for professional mixed martial arts and for professional basketball.

Exercise doesn't just help win games. It can increase your life expectancy by preventing or reversing arthritis, osteoporosis, obesity, loss of muscle mass (sarcopenia), age-related loss of function, diabetes, and cardiovascular diseases. And it improves sleep, mood, metabolism, physical appearance, libido, and creativity.

When I'm talking to investor groups, I tell them about the mechanical steroid for a special reason. The best way to get richer, after all, is to live longer and allow the power of exponential portfolio growth to do its magic.

I understand that it can be hard to find time to work out. It can also be frustrating when improvement is slow in coming, while joint pain and muscle soreness may arrive quickly, especially for those of us who are older.

Until I started using the device several years ago, I felt my efforts at exercise were only slowing my descent into age-related frailty, and slow failure is never fun. But since integrating this thermoregulatory device into my workouts, I've increased my flexibility, strength, and endurance. I look forward to every workout and start planning the next one as soon I've finished the last.

Mammalian Thermoregulation

The story of the mechanical steroid begins with Stanford biologists Dr. Craig Heller and Dr. Dennis Grahn.[32]   The two professors are the world's leading authorities on mammalian thermoregulation, the processes by which a mammal strives for an optimal body temperature.

For decades, Heller and Grahn studied how hibernating mammals maintain a steady core body temperature in freezing cold as well as in intense heat. Using implanted sensors and infrared photography, they solved a long-standing medical puzzle.

In the palms of your hands (or, if you're a bear, in the palms of your paws) as well as in the soles of your feet and in your cheeks are densely packed masses of veins called *retia venosa*. They are capable of quickly swelling to increase the volume of blood they carry by about 14-fold.[33]

These masses of veins present an evolutionary puzzle. What survival advantage offsets the obvious disadvantage of packing veins so near the surface of the body, where they are exposed to a higher risk of cuts or other trauma that could produce severe bleeding?

Heller and Grahn solved the puzzle by studying bears and other well-insulated hibernating animals. Infrared photography of bears detected heat being vented from the pads in their paws as well as their snouts. Humans share the same system for rapid heat dissipation.

---

32 Grahn is a senior research scientist in the Biological Sciences Department at Stanford University. Heller, former chairman of the Biological Sciences Department at Stanford and former chairman of the Defense Advanced Research Projects Agency (DARPA), is the coauthor of a widely used biology text.
33 See http://www.biomedcentral.com/1471-2377/8/14.

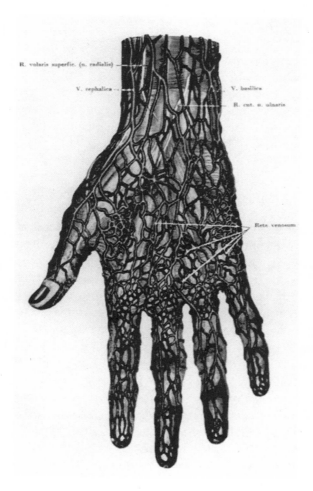

Further research found that all mammals, including humans, have a supplementary circulatory system that kicks in when the temperature of the body's core rises. Arterial blood is rerouted away from the general capillary system that handles oxygen and nutrition delivery and toward the retia venosa—the radiators—in your palms and other extremities.

The veins of the retia venosa swell to many times their resting size to enable venting of excess heat. As you radiate heat, cooled blood flows directly back to the heart and protects the vulnerable brain and other organs, including the heart itself, from being damaged by overheating.

Meet the Wall

This is a marvelous cooling system, of course, but its function is so important for protecting your brain and other organs from permanent damage that it is accompanied by back-up mechanisms. Without that back-up, vigorous exercise might overwhelm the retia venosa, which can only radiate heat so fast. Then very bad things would happen, starting with heat stroke.

One of the safety mechanisms sits in the brain itself. When you are in danger of overheating, the brain makes exertion extremely difficult and unpleasant. You may try to contract muscles at maximum force, but your brain won't send the signals to do it.

Other defenses operate in the muscle cells. As blood is routed away from limbs to protect the core, the normal flow of nutrients and oxygen to the muscle cells is cut off. Heat and waste materials, such as lactic acid and carbon dioxide, build up. Then the mitochondria that convert food into usable energy shut down, because an enzyme they need (pyruvate kinase) won't function at above a certain temperature. So muscle cells run out of power and stop producing more heat. It's a natural fail-safe mechanism.

These responses to overheating may seem dire, but it you are an active person, they have saved your life many times. When you've done a serious workout, you "hit the wall," which is your body's way of halting dangerously excessive heat production.

What's good for your core organs, however, can be hard on muscle and connective tissues, which are second-class citizens in the hierarchy of your body's priorities. While critical organs are being protected, muscle and connective tissues "slow cook" until healthy core temperature and normal circulation are restored.

Delayed-onset muscle soreness is one result of this heat buildup, but it's by no means the most serious. If you hit the wall often and hard enough, you can cancel the health benefits of working out. Extreme overtraining also cripples the immune system.

So we have to walk the corridor between too little exercise and too much. One way to keep within the corridor and still achieve rapid muscle growth is to use anabolic steroids, which promote protein synthesis and recovery. Steroids, however, can cause trouble—which in men may be shrinkage of the testicles, reduced sperm count or infertility, hair loss, or the growth of breast tissue. Women may grow facial hair, suffer male-pattern baldness, disruption or halting of menstrual cycles and enlargement of the clitoris.

A less troublesome alternative to chemical steroids is to rapidly cool the body's core during and immediately after exercise. That allows the blood to resume its normal circulation through muscle and connective tissues. Excess heat is cleared out within minutes, and mitochondrial energy production promptly resumes, accelerating the repair of cells. The flow of oxygen and nutrients returns to muscles and connective tissues, while waste gases and other products are quickly cleared.

In short, with rapid cooling, vigorous exercise promotes adaptive strengthening while the related stress and damage, as well as the associated pain, are minimized. The capacity to exercise goes up, and recovery is much more rapid. The gains available from exercise are greatly increased.

This is not just theory. It is clinically validated reality and an example of how biological discoveries are yielding new health technologies.

The story of how Heller and Grahn made it happen is fascinating.

Beat the Wall

Once they discovered how the body unloads excess heat, they began to wonder if they could give the process a little help.

First, they knew they could drain heat from the core by running cold water over the hands—a practice common among summertime construction workers. They learned that another effective method is to put the palm in contact with a perfusion pad, which is a soft, enclosed network of tubes filled with cold water. The big breakthrough, though, came with the aid of electronic sensors and computerized data collection. They discovered that subjecting the palm to a slight vacuum caused the veins in the retia venosa to expand even further and give up heat much, much faster.

They were interested initially in medical applications for their new technology but later recognized how it could amplify the benefits of physical exercise.

The device they developed, called AVAcore CoreControl, has two parts, the first of which holds ice water, a pump, and a microchip to control water temperature and vacuum pressure. The second part is a glove that seals around one hand. In it, water at the optimal temperature passes through a perfusion pad in contact with the palm.

Even after intense exercise, the device takes only a few minutes to restore normal core temperature, not the hours an unaided body would need. Cellular damage is minimized and recovery is accelerated dramatically. It works with both resistance training and cardiovascular workouts.

The strength and endurance gained can be maintained through unaided exercise, even if you stop using the device.

AVAcore's benefits are particularly important for older people, whose thermoregulatory abilities have declined with age and who suffer joint and flexibility problems. Restoring youthful blood flow to the joints and ligaments strengthens them. In my own experience, I'm now doing exercises that, because of joint problems, I wasn't able to do several years ago.

I believe thermoregulatory augmentation is *the* most important advancement in fitness technology since the ancient Greeks pioneered progressive training.

Chapter 26

Changing the Odds at the Big Casino

W hile I love what thermoregulation has done for me personally, it delivers only a little of what most people are hoping for from biotech. In fact, I'll tell you what tops the public's wish list: the conquest of cancer and heart disease, which together account for about half of all deaths in the US.

Let's start with cancer.

I remember a piece, probably from the American Cancer Society, which aired on television when I was three or four years old. It showed a stark, black-and-white picture of five people sitting around a dinner table as a grim voice-over announced, "One in five people will die of cancer."

I had two siblings, and I was old enough to count, so I knew that my family totaled five. To my young mind, the message meant that one of us was about to die. For days, I was consumed with dread. Finally, I talked to my mother, a registered nurse, about what I had heard. She explained a few things about statistics, somewhat reducing my stress. Sixty years later, however, it's still true that one in five dies of cancer.

It's not that we haven't made any progress in the war on cancer (we have), but today people live much longer than when I was a child, and cancer rates rise with age. However, while the odds of surviving a cancer have improved, the rate of cancer mortality has remained remarkably stable. For that reason, simply hearing the C-word from your doctor can be an overwhelming experience. Of course, this could be said of any fatal disease, such as Alzheimer's or Parkinson's, but for most of us, cancer carries a special terror.

First, cancer is unpredictable. It can show up at any time, anywhere, and for no apparent reason. One slang term for the disease I've heard since I was a kid, "the big casino," reflects this. Without a substantial understanding of cellular biology, talking about cancer is tantamount to talking about a curse,

145

which is exactly how some pre-modern societies viewed the disease.

Cancer invades your body and refuses to leave. It isn't static; it evolves as the immune system attempts to fight it. In many ways, cancer proceeds as though it were a malevolent or alien intelligence, and it comes in many varieties. Exacerbating the curse of cancer, today's standard treatments can be just as harmful as the cancer itself. Right now, the only way to destroy cancer is to damage ourselves along with it.

Cancer should also be a scary word for investors. Treatments are in development that will be orders of magnitude more effective than anything available today. Investors betting on marginal improvements in old technology could take a hit. When fully licensed, even one of these new therapies could leave the old cancer treatment industry in shambles.

Because I'm in touch with some of the sharpest people waging the fight against cancer, I'm convinced that we are on the verge of dramatically improving that "one in five" mortality stat, perhaps bringing it close to zero. For this reason, I approach investing in old-style cancer-related companies with great caution.

Some morning in the not-so-distant future, a press release from a biotech startup is going to tell the world that cancer, as we knew it, is over. At that point, the $100 billion cancer industry will implode. Companies, even in the realm of Big Pharma, will collapse, and a lot of investors are going to be in pain—although their chances of out-living the pain will have gone way up.

Not long ago, we caught a glimpse of that morning when a 49-year-old woman with severe breast cancer received a new treatment at Memorial Sloan Kettering Cancer Center. The dramatic results generated headlines like *Forbes*' "Immune System Drugs Melt Tumors in New Study, Leading a Cancer Revolution."[34] I'm not sure that this therapy is "leading" the revolution, but a revolution is underway.[35]

The therapy used two drugs that had already been used separately, a compound called Opdivo that protects T cells and a monoclonal antibody called Yervoy that blocks cancer's ability to turn off a critical component of the immune system.

Last year, equally stunning results were reported for Juno Therapeutics' chimeric antigen receptor (CAR) T-cell therapy. Of twenty-seven patients

34 http://www.forbes.com/sites/matthewherper/2015/04/20/immune-system-drugs-melt-tumors-leading-a-cancer-revolution/
35 More details can be found in the *New England Journal of Medicine*. See http://www.nejm.org/doi/full/10.1056/NEJMoa1414428?query=featured_home

with refractory acute lymphoblastic leukemia, twenty-four went into remission, six of whom continued to appear disease-free a year later. Billions of dollars of capitalization have flown into Juno Therapeutics, Kite Pharma, and other companies working on CAR T-cell therapies.[36]

Thinking as an investor, I'm cool on these companies because, despite huge successes, I don't think they're going to win the race, at least not for long. Moreover, their drugs are extremely expensive, some with six-figure price tags.

For the next several years, I expect constant tumult in the cancer drug business, as important but incremental improvements are announced. It's going to be a very dangerous investment environment. It might be profitable for fleet-footed traders, but I'm much more interested in the long-term transformational winners.

Let's take some time to review the science.

Cells That Forget to Die

Every minute of every day, quadrillions of processes go on in your roughly 100 trillion cells. Cells are constantly dying and being replaced. Some types of cells (e.g. heart, eyes, and kidneys) survive longer than others (e.g., skin, hair, and stomach lining), but of all the cells that were in your body seven years ago, almost none are alive today. Their replacements have filled in.

How long a cell lasts and why some live longer than others is determined by the telomeres of its chromosomes. Telomeres work like the plastic tips on the end of shoelaces that prevent them from fraying and falling apart— they are located at the end a cell's chromosomes, and except in the first few days of life, every time a normal cell divides, it uses up a telomere.

Over the course of a lifetime, you run down your stock of telomeres. The shorter the telomere strands at the ends of your chromosomes get, the more prone to error and mutation the DNA replication process becomes. Some of the mutations that occur become cancers. Currently, the most promising strategy for halting this literally dead-end process is to switch out old cells and replace them with rejuvenated cells carrying full telomere strands.

---

36 Here's a good overview from the National Cancer Institute: http://www.cancer.gov/about-cancer/treatment/research/car-t-cells

Several stem cell therapies based on this strategy are being developed and will probably launch first in Japan, where regulators—faced with a rapidly aging population—operate with a sense of urgency about life-extending therapies. Until such therapies are available, though, your telomere strands will continue inexorably to shorten.

Fortunately, our immune system constantly monitors the cells of our body. If a mutation causes a cell to become dysfunctional, that cell will be signaled to initiate apoptosis, or cell suicide.

Somewhat counter-intuitively, cell suicide is critical for a healthy body and for your survival. If a cell's continued growth and replication would cause more harm than good to the organism, it should "volunteer" for apoptosis.[37]

Information Standoff

I have some good news and some bad news.

The bad news is that, right now, you have cancer. In fact, you developed about a million cancer cells today.

The good news is that your immune system will get rid of today's one-million cancers, just as it did with yesterday's one-million cancers.

Every human being develops cancer every single day. This may seem impossible, given how deadly cancer can be, but it's true. Normally, your immune system identifies and destroys cancer cells as quickly as they appear. Cancer cells are formidable opponents, but fortunately, your immune system has the better team. Over the course of a lifespan, you vanquish cancer billions of times.

But it's not enough to dominate the season—you must win every single game. A single loss by the T cells to a developing cancer puts you in grave danger. None of your previous victories will matter a bit if you get that one-in-a-billion case that your immune system fails to dispatch in time.

The presence of cancer doesn't mean your immune system has shut down. It simply means the cancer has found a way to fool your immune system or hide from it.

---

37 Apoptosis is also critical for fetal development. Without it, we would still be equipped with the webbed hands and toes, as well as the tails, we all had as fetuses. Though the tail might actually be cool, the destruction of unneeded individual cells allows the fetus to live and grow.

Understanding this fact is revolutionizing oncology. More and more scientists advocate treatments that train the immune system to wise up to cancer's tricks. Instead of firing the immune system team, bring in a specialized coach.

Helping the immune system win the biological information battle is what makes a treatment successful. It restores the immune system's ability to seek out and destroy damaged cells as they emerge.

Chapter 27

Cancer Treatments: From Double-Edged Swords to Magic Bullets

A cancer must do everything just right to take root in the body, but once it has latched on, it can be hard to stop. In many cases, such as with prostate and lymphatic cancers, the conventional strategy is to lose the battle as slowly as possible and hope to keep the patient alive until something else kills him.

In the near future, though, we'll look back at this attitude as medical barbarism.

The weapons we use to fight cancer today are highly effective cell killers. They are so strong and so dangerous, in fact, that they kill noncancerous cells as well. They're double-edged swords. They damage the patient almost as much as they damage the cancer, which is why much of the advance in chemotherapy amounts to improved deftness in selecting the chemical and the dose.

While development of treatments based on the cellular processes that drive cancer is already well advanced, the only cancer-removal methods in general use today still are surgery, radiation, and chemotherapy. Each has problems.

Surgery hasn't changed much from the procedures of the ancient Greeks and Romans. They used anesthetics and disinfectants, and many of their surgical instruments are remarkably similar to what you'll find in a "modern" hospital. They also recognized thousands of years ago that surgery wasn't always effective against mysteries like cancer.

The scalpel is still not the ideal tool for the oncologist. If a single invisible cancer cell is left behind, it may migrate and start a new tumor elsewhere in the body. Moreover, the trauma of major surgery further

151

weakens the patient.

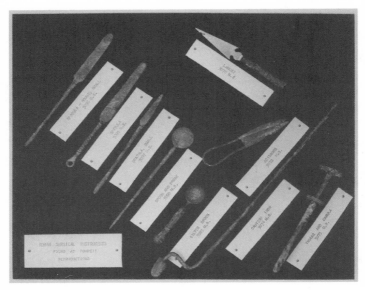

Ancient Roman surgical tools found at Pompeii, from Otis Historical Archives,
National Museum of Health and Medicine (source: Wikimedia Commons)

Radiation, while a far more modern treatment, can be just as damaging as surgery. After the first observations of X-ray radiation in 1895, attempts were made to enlist it for treating tuberculosis, lupus, epithelioma and other medical conditions. Radium, a radioactive element first identified by Marie Curie, was widely used in medicine until researchers realized that the human tolerance for radiation had been vastly overestimated. Curie herself carried tubes of radium in the pockets of her lab coat and ultimately died from the exposure.

Radiation therapy often is unsuccessful. The cure rate for head and neck cancers is only 23%.

Chemotherapy, the newest of the three pillars of oncology, was developed in the 1940s from components of WWI mustard gas. Doctors studying chemical warfare agents noticed that they stopped the division of some somatic cells and realized they might do the same to cancer cells. This was a breakthrough, but as I've already pointed out and as doctors soon observed, chemotherapy also damages noncancerous cells, although their tolerance is generally higher.

Melting Cancer from Within

Several revolutionary approaches to dealing with cancer have emerged from recent discoveries about the nature of cancer cells. I hope you'll understand why I can't name all the companies that are moving these technologies forward. The investors who fund my research have paid for access to that information and wouldn't be happy if I simply gave it away to everyone. But I can give you a few examples.

Bexion Pharmaceuticals is a private company with a drug candidate that could demolish the old cancer treatment model.

The Bexion story started in 2002 at Cincinnati Children's Hospital Medical Center, when a researcher, Xiaoyang Qi, PhD., noticed that the surfaces of the tumor cells he was studying always seemed to carry low levels of the protein saposin C (or SapC). If a cell is healthy, on the other hand, SapC won't be found loitering on its surface although it will be present inside a healthy cell's lysosomes.

Yeah. Lysosomes. Stay with me. Learning about lysosomes is worth it.

Lysosomes are the most bizarre of our organelles. Organelles, as the name implies, are tiny organ-like structures found within individual cells. The cell's nucleus (which contains the cell's DNA) and the cell's energy-producing mitochondria are other examples of organelles.

When I think of lysosomes, I'm reminded of the acid-blooded monster in the Ridley Scott film *Alien*. That fictional creature can digest anything and, if injured, spouts powerful acidic fluids that destroy everything around it. Lysosomes are its microscopic equivalent, and they operate inside nearly every cell in your body.

Lysosomes produce and contain acids and enzymes capable of destroying anything troublesome they encounter in the cell. Normally, they patrol the cell they occupy and break down stuff that doesn't belong there, such as viruses and parts of the cell that have worn out. When it's time for the cell itself to go away (because it's worn or damaged) the lysosomes open up and dump their acidic contents and their SapC, digesting the entire cell from the inside out. This is what cell suicide, or apoptosis, looks like up close.

This climactic event is triggered by increased levels of the chemical *ceramide*. Part of a cancer cell's survival strategy is to disable its own suicide switch by converting ceramide into another chemical, called *sphingosine*. As a survival bonus, the cancer cell can use the sphingosine for a number of mischievous purposes, including promoting its own blood supply, resisting anti-cancer drugs, and dispatching tumor cells to colonize other locations in the body.

Assuming you agree that cancer is a bad thing, it would be a good thing to find a way to block a cancer cell's ability to transform ceramide into sphingosine. Many scientists have tried and all have failed.[38]

So, back to SapC, a protein found in the acid-bleeding lysosomes of all cells and at low concentrations on the surfaces of tumors. When Dr. Qi noticed free SapC around tumors, he wondered whether it *caused* cells to turn cancerous. But when he exposed healthy cells to SapC, no cancers developed.

Qi explained his puzzlement to a colleague, who suggested boosting the levels of SapC around a culture of cancer cells, to see what might happen. When the protein was added to cancer cell cultures in sufficient concentrations, the cancer cells melted away.[39]

This led to the launch of Bexion Pharmaceuticals. While Bexion found SapC enormously promising as a stand-alone cancer drug, delivering it with a *nanovesicle* technology made it even more effective. The delivery vehicle was a micro-tube built out of a lipid (fatty) molecule, DOPS[40] , found in the human body.

I learned about the SapC—DOPS technology from Dr. Cameron Durrant, a brilliant scientist and former Big Pharma executive. At the time, all that researchers knew for sure was that all kinds of tumors in test animals, even brain tumors, seemed to melt away when exposed to SapC-DOPS -- but it wasn't clear why. Since then, Bexion CEO and President Ray Takigiku has pieced together a picture of how the drug works.

Apoptotic Mimicry

Right now, your body includes millions of cells that have identified themselves as abnormal and are raising their ceramide levels to prompt their lysosomes to dump their acidic cargo.

---

38 Other scientists have proposed that it might be possible to create a bioweapon capable of increasing ceramide levels to activate the lysosomes' cell suicide function throughout the body. This ceramide weapon would cause human targets to melt.

39 The SapC added to the cultures was accompanied by dioleoylphosphatidylserine. The role of the latter substance is unknown.

40 DOPS is short for dioleoylphosphatidylserine.

Given your nonstop supply of abnormal cells, you might wonder why your ever vigilant immune system doesn't exhaust itself attacking them. The simple answer is that it doesn't need to, since the abnormal cells are already setting themselves up for death, and as they do, they post a "Don't bother with me" sign by spreading a particular molecule, phosphatidylserine (PS), on their exterior.

Cancers trick the immune system by painting PS on their own cell surfaces and thereby masquerading as dying apoptotic cells.[41] That's how they stay alive. SapC gives them a second chance to die.

SapC Targets PS on Tumor Cells

SapC molecules are always found around tumors but never around normal cells. On a molecular level, the reason for this is clear. In acidic conditions and only in acidic conditions, SapC tends to fuse with PS (the death-notice molecule that a tumor fraudulently presents on its surface)— and acidic conditions are characteristic of tumors but not of normal cells.

SapC is part of our natural defense against cancer. Once it has fused with the PS on a cancer cell's surface, it metabolizes elements of the membrane into ceramides that promote cell suicide. In other words, SapC tries to overcome the cancer's ability to block production of suicide-inducing ceramide. In the early stages of a cancer, natural levels of SapC may succeed at this.

Later, after a cancer has become well established, natural levels of SapC won't be sufficient to tip the ceramide balance toward the cancer's destruction. That's when a combination of SapC and DOPS is needed to convert elements in the cell membrane to ceramides on a scale big enough to be lethal.

---

41 In moving PS to the outside of the cell, as theatrical make-up to impersonate a dying apoptotic cell, a cancer accomplishes other molecular mischief. It triggers an inflammation process that promotes the production of proteins that block apoptosis. And it stimulates the production of vascular endothelial factor, which promotes the rapid development of blood vessels to support the tumor and its growth.

Cancer cells also use PS to build exosomes (micro packages) containing cancer DNA. When shed by a cancer cell, the exosomes can travel to transform healthy cells into cancer cells. Because they're built from molecules signaling that a cell is dead, the exosomes elude the immune system and are free to roam and convert.

SapC-DOPS kills tumor cells with astonishing speed, but it is harmless to all other cells. This has been confirmed both in cell cultures and in animals infected with human tumors, including brain tumors. If it works as well as many scientists expect, it could change cancer treatment completely— no more surgery, no more radiation, no more chemotherapy.

Interestingly, the only type of cancer that SapC-DOPS doesn't seem to kill is non-tumor cancers, which don't need an acidic environment. Blood cancers are the obvious examples. Fortunately, a number of immunotherapies are on track for treating non-acidic cancers.

Chapter 28

Nipping Cancer in the Bud

T he meaning of *vaccine* has expanded considerably during our lifetimes. Third-generation vaccines have practically nothing to do with the vaccines most of us were given when we were children.
Edward Jenner's discovery that a weakened virus could teach the immune system to fight the virus's more damaging cousins has been applied to control polio, smallpox, and other infectious diseases. Long after Jenner, scientists learned to develop safer vaccines when they discovered that a specific component of a virus, an antigen, could trigger a full response from the immune system. Such antigen-only vaccines now protect against diphtheria and hepatitis B.

Today's vaccine technology can do even more. It can, for example, train your immune system to fight cancer.

DNA Vaccines

The DNA in your genome is not the only DNA you have. Most cells (red blood cells are the prominent exception) contain mitochondria, the organelles that process glucose into ready-to-use biochemical energy. Each liver cell holds thousands of mitochondria. Other cell types hold only a few.

Each mitochondrion carries multiple rings of DNA, each with the same 37 protein-encoding genes. Similar rings are found in bacteria (which supports the belief that mitochondria are descended from bacteria). Your mitochondrial DNA is completely different from the DNA in your genome. It is much simpler, and it came to you solely from your mother. Its method for producing proteins also is different.

A gene manufactures a protein through transcription, a process that, when triggered in the central genome, takes place only on a specific section of a chromosome, with specific starting and ending points. The cool thing about protein manufacture with DNA rings, whether in mitochondria or in bacteria, is that it can run continuously.

Gene transcription in the nucleus is like getting on a complex highway system and going from point A to point B, making the components of a protein along the way. Ring protein production, on the other hand, is like a closed-loop model railroad with an endlessly repeating process.

This nonstop operation offers genetic engineers a powerful drug-producing mechanism. They modify bacterial DNA by adding genes that will produce the therapeutic proteins they want. The altered DNA rings can then be inserted into a body's cells and activated, so that the body produces its own medicine.

Such DNA vaccines can include genes that produce specific antigens that train the immune system to look for and eliminate diseased cells. A mixture of such antigens can trigger a much wider range of immune responses than traditional vaccines. The ability to engineer proteins that the human body can produce for itself will prove far more valuable than just fighting cancers, however. DNA vaccines can also be used to boost production of chemicals whose supply normally declines with aging... but I'll get to that later.

Experimental DNA vaccines have already proven effective against viral, bacterial, and parasitic diseases, including malaria, and have demonstrated the ability to attack cancers. Even at the low doses used in safety trials, this technology produces measurable benefits.

Dendritic Cell-Based Vaccines

The new immunotherapeutics use only part of a virus or other pathogen to teach the immune system to recognize and attack the entire pathogen. This is the same strategy the immune system itself uses.

T cells are the soldiers of the immune system—some gather intelligence, others engage in direct combat with the enemy or tell the immune system when a battle has been won. Just like real soldiers, though, the front-line T cells need training.

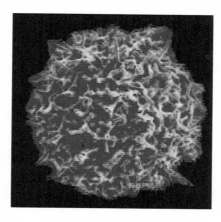

"Healthy Human T Cell" by NIAID/NIH - NIAID Flickr's photostream. Licensed under Public Domain via Wikimedia Commons

All T cells are born in the marrow of our large bones, but at that point, they're "naïve," meaning they haven't yet learned to carry out specialized tasks. Specialization, or maturation, takes place when an immature T cell migrates to the thymus (which is where the T in T cells comes from).

The thymus gland, located between the heart and the sternum, processes and stores information about threats to the body delivered to it by specialized T cells. If you have an acquired immunity, your thymus has stored the information needed to quickly train naïve T cells to recognize and fight the respective disease.[42]

Whether a pathogen is an invading virus or a cancer, a successful response from the immune system starts with building a profile of the enemy.

Special intelligence-gathering cells called *antigen-presenting cells* (APCs) roam the body, constantly searching for signs of a threat. When the APCs find a trouble-maker, they capture antigens from it and pass them to

---

42 The T might also stand for tonsils, as these lymphoid organs in the throat, once thought vestigial and useless, also prepare T cells for battle.

The fact that researchers have only recently begun to verify that tonsils are part of the adaptive immune system is yet another sign of the accelerating pace of biological discovery—the biotech singularity. New understanding about tonsils may, in fact, have consequences because the thymus shrinks as we age. At puberty, it weighs about 35 grams, but after the age of 70, in most people only about 5 grams.

immune system combat cells, as though they were letting a hound dog sniff at a fugitive's left-behind sock. Based on this antigen "intel," the immune system develops specialized weapons (antibodies) to destroy the threat.

The most common type of intel-gathering APCs are dendritic cells. They figure out how to find pathogens and, after analyzing them, move critical antigen information to their surfaces to share with the rest of the immune system.

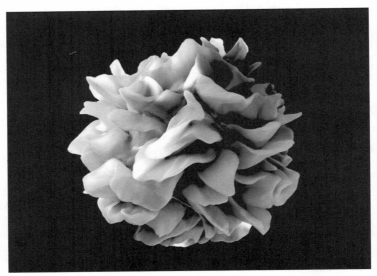

Artistic rendering of dendritic cell by National Institutes of Health (NIH) via Wikipedia

Cancers happen, so it's obvious that our biological homeland-security systems aren't perfect. Scientists are discovering ways to strengthen them. One of the most exciting is the engineering of dendritic cells to present antigens that a cancer is carrying but that the natural dendritic cells have overlooked.

While this approach has worked in the lab, it is extremely expensive—a price tag close to six figures. And producing the engineered dendritic cells requires time that an advanced-stage cancer patient may not have.

An alternative now being tested is a stem-cell-based vaccine that could be used off the shelf to treat anyone with cancer. That might seem impossible, given that cancer cells come in so many varieties and are constantly mutating. However, nearly all cancers share certain characteristics that, it is hoped, the immune system could be taught to recognize.

One of those badges of cancer is the movement of phosphatidylserines to the surface of the cancer cell. Another is immortalization.

It's bad enough that cancer cells replicate rapidly and can recruit other cells. But they are even more dangerous than that: they don't die. In fact, they don't even age. They accomplish this trick through "immortalization," just as embryonic stem cells do, via activation of the telomerase gene.

The telomerase gene is largely inactive in adult cells. In embryonic cells, iPS cells, and cancer cells, however, the gene is switched on. The cell's telomere thread is constantly replenished, and so the cell doesn't age. Cultures of embryonic and cancer cells can live for thousands of generations, unlike most cell lines, that die when they reach their Hayflick Limit of 120 or so replications.

The activated telomerase gene is a target for the new generation of vaccines. One strategy is to reconstitute the patient's dendritic cells to flag telomerase as an antigen. Once the immune system is trained to attack cells that exhibit telomerase, it will kill cancer cells. The technology to make such vaccines has been validated in human trials.

P53 Tumor Suppressor Gene

The genetic mechanisms that orchestrate and protect a cell's life also guard the genome itself. One source of protection for the genome is controlled by the p53 gene.[43]

Chromosome strands are fragile. They can be broken by cosmic rays, viruses, and other micro-hooligans. When a break is detected, a protein assembled by the p53 gene activates a process that may rejoin the broken strand. But if the damage entails a potentially dangerous rearrangement of genes that might lead to a tumor, the process will force the cell to shut down. In other words, the p53 strategy for dealing with a cell with a broken chromosome is fix it or kill it.

Normally, humans inherit the gene from both parents. However, if either of those copies is defective or missing,[44] the individual is nearly certain to

---

43 http://www.genecards.org/cgi-bin/carddisp.pl?gene=TP53
44 The condition is known as Li-Fraumeni syndrome

develop cancer.

A mutated p53 gene is found in about half of all cancers. In other cancers, the p53 protein's anti-tumor mechanisms are being blocked, even though the gene itself is functioning. In either case, for a cancer to survive, it must sabotage or elude p53's function (which is to repair or shut down mutated cells).

The protein assembled by the p53 gene once was believed to cause cancer. Now it is seen as a tumor suppressor that in normal cells activates the production of DNA-repair proteins. When necessary, it can stop cell replication and induce cell suicide.

Much effort has gone into to reactivating normal p53 functioning in cancer cells. One method seems to work, with strong pre-clinical data in leukemia, pancreatic, breast, lung, colon, prostate, and HPV-induced cancers. Several human trials are underway.

Galectin-3s and the Emergence of Glycoscience

While some big biomedical topics, such as the Alzheimer's-related buildup of amyloid plaques in the brain, have gained public attention, many new discoveries about disease and aging haven't. Nonetheless, biotech revolutions are happening, even if they escape widespread notice. The science of galectin-3 proteins is a perfect example.

Galectin-3 proteins[45] control a variety of biological functions, including wound repair. But as our bodies age, these helpers are increasingly likely to become trouble makers.

Galectin-3s gone wrong may block drug-induced apoptosis in tumor cancers, which is bad enough. In addition, tumors secrete galectin-3 proteins that kill the T cells that should be detecting and killing the tumors.

The problem may stem from galectin-3s' role in protecting newly forming scar tissue from attack by the immune system. Tumors use galectin-3s to gain the same kind of protection. They wrap themselves in a filmy web of gal-3s that is lethal to T cells that touch it.

A brilliant Russian scientist noticed that the shape of the galectin-3 molecule was similar to certain plant sugars he had studied. He hypothesized

---

45 Galectin-3 proteins are assembled by the LGALS3 gene.

that these harmless plant sugars, similar to those you eat every day, might also bind to T cells and occupy all the spots where galectin-3s produced by cancers might attach and attack.

He linked the plant sugar molecules to a common chemotherapeutic and then tested the material in cancer-bearing lab mice. The results were nearly miraculous. Not only did the mice recover from cancer completely, they seemed untroubled by the therapy. In fact, their livers and kidneys, which likely would have been tormented by conventional chemo, were healthy.

In cell cultures, we've seen T cells that were dying from galectin-3-induced apoptosis resurrected by these plant-sugar drugs. Apparently the plant sugars bind so strongly with the surface of T cells that they elbow the lethal galectin-3 proteins out of the way. Thus protected, the T cells then attack the cancer cells and destroy them.

This sweet chemo technology is now going through clinical trials.

Next-Generation Diagnostics

Early detection of cancer boosts the success rate of conventional therapies. Early detection combined with the new therapies will reduce most cancers to minor annoyances. The most promising development in early detection technology is large-scale gene expression testing.

With its mutated DNA, each type of cancer cell produces a characteristic set of proteins not present in healthy cells. Cancer cells leak these gene-assembled proteins, which are markers for disease. Every one of those markers can be detected via blood and even urine testing, but there are thousands to look for.

A new device that screens for all of them at once is built from a glass plate with a large array of tiny hollows, each holding a reactant sensitive to a specific protein. These microarrays (called biochips if built with electronics that communicate results), can be tailored to test for as many different proteins as necessary. Such massive-scale testing for protein markers not only detects the presence of cancer, it often identifies the type of cancer, its stage of development, where it is located, and where it originated.

The first such testing systems, which use standard protein arrays available in most clinical laboratories, are aimed at specific types of cancers—but that will change soon.

Within a few years, we'll see universal cancer tests that cost no more than a standard single-cancer test (such as the prostate-specific antigen (PSA) screening) costs today. And they will be far more accurate, with few false positives. Being inexpensive, the tests will be part of routine checkups and will detect cancers long before any damage has been done. I say this with confidence because the technologies already exist.

Chapter 29

Rampant Killers:
Virus-Borne Diseases

The Ebola epidemic in 2014 claimed more victims than any prior outbreak of this particularly gruesome disease. The virus damages cells so badly that victims may bleed from every opening of the body. Depending on the level of care they receive, 50% to 90% of those who contract the virus die.

As the virus began to spread across national borders, media coverage resembled trailers for horror movies. Tom Frieden, head of the US Centers for Disease Control and Prevention, told a House subcommittee that Ebola would inevitably come to America. US border patrol agents, already stressed to control tuberculosis and other diseases coming in from Mexico, began to worry about the arrival of Ebola from Africa. In the UK, border agents threatened to go on strike unless flights from infected regions were halted.

Predictably, a lot of people demanded that "somebody do something" to help Ebola victims.

Before the outbreak, Western pharmaceutical companies were often accused of using third-world patients as guinea pigs. During the outbreak, we heard that Western drug makers were greedy hoarders for not making experimental drugs available to the developing world. Some Africans reacted with resentment when two American missionaries were given access to ZMapp, a monoclonal antibody drug under development by Mapp Biopharmaceutical of San Diego. Dr. Tolbert Nyenswah, Liberia's assistant health minister, told the *Wall Street Journal*, "The population here is asking: 'You said there was no cure for Ebola, but the Americans are curing it?'"

Also predictably, regulators responded by loosening the rules on using Ebola drug candidates. In particular, the FDA lifted the hold it had placed only weeks before on clinical testing of a drug by Canada-based Tekmira

Pharmaceuticals, which uses a short sequence of RNA to block the action of target genes. In this case, the drug interfered with the Ebola viruses' ability to reproduce.

I don't want to demonize the people at the FDA. Nevertheless, it's helpful to ask why it made sense one week to halt an Ebola drug's progression toward approval because of marginal safety concerns... and the next week, to put the drug on a fast track toward approval.

As much as the FDA adapted to public sentiment, the World Health Organization (WHO), which controls the transfer of experimental drugs across national borders, eased up on developers of Ebola drugs.

From one week to the next, nothing had changed—except public opinion. There was no new scientific knowledge. Regulators couldn't even honestly say they were surprised by the outbreak. They knew it was coming, just not when. Anybody who is familiar with Ebola knows its cyclical pattern. So if the risk/reward calculation justifies the easing of regulatory hurdles when an inevitable outbreak occurs, the same calculation should have applied before it occurs.

If you're reading this from the relative security of a Western country, you might think that regulatory schizophrenia doesn't threaten you. If so, I'd like to walk you through a thought experiment that might change your mind.

Ebola, like every other virus type, produces trillions of mutants every day. Imagine that one of those Ebola mutations helps the lucky virus survive in the air. Ebola has become an airborne disease that can be spread by sneezing.

Suppose it then starts killing at an annual rate of a quarter-million people worldwide, including 40,000 Americans each year. Do you think politicians and regulators would finally stop dragging their feet on drug approvals, which under current rules cost hundreds of millions of dollars and a decade or longer to complete? Would the paradigm shift from avoiding remote, hypothetical risks of drug side effects to unleashing companies that can deliver effective treatments?

Now let's raise the stakes. Suppose virologists point out that this new strain of Ebola is likely to undergo further mutations and eventually kill many millions of people in pandemics on the scale of the Black Death. Do you think regulators would drop the practice of waging years-long arguments over warning labels and let doctors start using every promising Ebola drug?

The answer is yes, of course.   But the hypothetical menace of Ebola I just described actually fits a real, existing virus. It is a far greater threat to mankind—and to you personally—than Ebola. It's influenza.

So why are Ebola drug candidates given a warmer regulatory welcome than influenza drugs? Science has nothing to do with it. Epidemiology has nothing to do with it. The principles of public health have nothing to do with it. Ebola drugs get fast-track treatment because the word "Ebola" strikes fear, while "flu" is a public communication ho-mum.

How to Eradicate Influenza

Influenza has already killed millions. Moreover, every virologist and epidemiologist knows that a truly terrifying mutation of a flu virus is evolving right now in the wild. It will put millions of people in the grave, hitting medical professionals hardest, and it will knock global gross domestic product (GDP) down by three to five points. It's coming, and there's nothing we can do about it.

Oh, wait. That's not quite right. There are, in fact, steps that would bring remarkable new influenza drugs, some already in development, to market faster. We're just not taking those steps. But we will when the pandemic hits, just as we've seen with Ebola. Unfortunately, at that point, the body count will already be in six figures, and it may be too late to avoid deaths on the scale of a major war.

There are scientists and investors who look to the future with clear eyes. These extraordinary individuals are working on transformational biotechnologies that will end influenza's lethal power in our lifetime.

Though the mainstream media rarely cover the pre-clinical work, that's where the game-changers come from. One is a never-before-seen category of drugs that combines biological signaling molecules with polymer delivery vehicles. The combo operates in the body like a fleet of submicroscopic machines.

If you read popular science magazines or watch science shows on TV, you've heard about a future when nanomachines will operate inside the body to fight disease. Those nonomachines aren't just in the future. Scientists are already building them. They start with astoundingly small, molecularly precise polymer shells, or vesicles. Then they attach large numbers of biological signaling molecules called ligands to the polymer vesicles.

Normally, a cell carries a characteristic set of ligands on its surface that act as signaling mechanisms for normal biological functions. The ligands work as selective docking mechanisms for proteins with complementary shapes. When a matching protein docks with a ligand, the event triggers an electrochemical signal, or pulse, capable of altering the shape, and thereby the function, of the ligand.

A virus exploits a cell's ligands to determine whether the cell would be a suitable host. The common influenza virus, for example, can replicate only inside a lung cell. When a flu virus finds a lung-cell ligand, it docks, and the resulting electrochemical signal allows it to enter. Once inside, the virus releases its payload and hijacks the cell's DNA-replicating mechanism to turn out copies of itself. When the load of virus particles gets big enough, they burst out of the cell and go on to infect other lung cells.

Scientists are now exploiting this ligand search, common to all viruses, by building tiny biomechanical killing machines that can float freely in the bloodstream and capture viruses like Venus flytraps. Taking the influenza virus as an example, scientists attach ligands associated with lung cells to submicroscopic polymer spheres. A single polymer vesicle can carry thousands of ligand molecules, which makes these structures far more attractive to circulating influenza viruses than lung cells that show only a few ligand docks.

When an influenza virus encounters one of these mechanisms, it docks with one of its ligands. The resulting electrochemical pulse causes the vesicle to open up, and the virus enters the vesicle just as it would a lung cell. There the virus releases its payload harmlessly and is permanently inactivated.

Unlike the conventional and only weakly effective anti-viral drugs that operate by interfering with virus replication, a ligand machine does direct, one-on-one battle with a virus. And because these nanoscale devices can't enter human cells, serious side effects are unlikely. In fact, the devices have demonstrated a remarkable lack of toxicity. In animal studies, the symptoms of many virus diseases disappear within hours.

Because ligand machines function independently of the host's biology, they likely will work in people just as well as they have in animals and in samples of human blood.

People will still want to get vaccinated against viral diseases, but we also will be able to directly attack viruses, from herpes and Ebola to shingles and influenza, after someone has been infected. And because the immune system doesn't recognize the polymers as bioactive pathogens, they linger in the bloodstream and continue to protect the patient from sickness, perhaps for months.

A few of the virus particles that get into the body will, however, manage to make their way into cells. So long as that happens on only a small scale, it actually helps the body by triggering a natural immune response.

Chapter 30

Superbugs and Antibiotic Armageddon

Viruses aren't the only "bugs" in our system. Hostile bacteria are another threat. To hear the mainstream media's current story about bacterial infection, we're all doomed. Deadly bacteria are becoming more and more resistant to antibiotics, and science will be helpless to deal with the apocalyptic threat. Oh, and the weatherman reports that the sky is falling.

As I write this chapter, the top search-engine returns on "superbug" include an NPR link titled "Antibiotics Can't Keep Up With 'Nightmare' Superbugs," a CBS News story called, "Superbugs: A ticking time bomb," and a BBC story warning that "Superbugs to kill 'more than cancer' by 2050." I recently watched part of a compelling British documentary called *Antibiotic Apocalypse*.

I'm not surprised by the end-of-the-world coverage. The story has everything needed for any journalist who yearns to report a problem so frightening that no one will object to the government stepping in to solve it.

Of course bacteria are developing immunity to all the antibiotics now in use, but there are other, revolutionary weapons against bacteria that will rescue mankind just as soon as they get past the regulatory roadblocks. Journalists seldom understand this. Rather, they focus on overuse of antibiotics by doctors and patients, which inevitably leads to demands for even more government regulation.

Despite the end-of-the-world headlines, the media line about antibiotic resistance is the biotech equivalent of peak oil. We're not running out of effective antibiotics any more than we are running out of fossil fuels. On the contrary, there is an entire new generation of antibiotics able to beat resistant strains of bacteria—as well as fungal and parasitic diseases—waiting to

171

come to market. These new drugs will not only kill the scariest "superbugs," they will solve the problem of bacterial resistance and solve it permanently.

Remarkable progress has been made toward using monoclonal antibodies and viruses to fight bacteria. I think the most interesting technology, however, is a mimic of the antibiotics your own body produces.

Why We Aren't Dead Already

Existing antibacterials attack infection in two steps. First they identify some molecule on the microorganism's surface and bind to it. Then, once attached, they transport a poison into the bacterium to disable or kill it.

But that's not the end of the story. Bacterial strains develop resistance by modifying the molecules that otherwise would attract an antibiotic, so that the drug can't recognize or bind to the bacteria. Bacteria also can modify their "efflux pumps" to expel the poison an antibiotic drug delivers.

The media cite the adaptive ability of bacteria to portray them as nearly invincible—the inevitable winners in their war with humans. The obvious problem with the story is that humans have always lived in a world teeming with bacteria.

In terms of total biomass, bacteria are the Earth's dominant life form. Your body is home to far more bacterial cells than human. While some of these "bugs" are symbiotic and support your health, others can cause serious disease. In fact, at this very moment, you are almost certainly carrying around some variety of the dreaded "flesh-eating bacteria."

So the question we should be asking is, "How do we all swim through this ocean of potentially deadly bacteria without succumbing?" That question led scientists to a whole new type of antibiotic that imitates the antimicrobial defenses we're born with. Found throughout the animal kingdom, including in insects, these natural antibiotics are called *defensins*.[46]

Defensins attach themselves electrostatically to bacteria and other microorganisms, including fungi and some viruses. For targeted microbes, this attachment is the hug of death. Defensins lock onto bacteria and other microorganisms and perforate their outer membranes. The resulting "leaks" disrupt the microorganisms' vital functions.

---

46 Structurally, defensins are peptides, short amino-acid chains with an electrostatic charge. (Larger amino-acid chains, by the way, are called proteins.)

Bacteria don't develop resistance to defensins. Whereas conventional antibiotics slip through a bacterium's cell wall and then disrupt the processes behind it, defensins rip holes in the wall itself. To escape the defensins, bacteria would have to develop entirely new outer-membrane characteristics, which these simple organisms aren't able to do.

Defensins are found in and on many human body parts, including the skin, tongue, cornea, salivary glands, kidneys, esophagus, and lungs. They form the protective barrier that prevents infection by ubiquitous bacteria. Only when this barrier is penetrated can infections occur.

Take, for example, the so-called flesh-eating bacteria, which cause *necrotizing fasciitis*. When the defensin barrier is intact, the bacteria responsible for necrotizing fasciitis are harmless, even if we're covered in them. But when the bacteria are allowed to bypass the defensin barrier, perhaps through a break in the skin, such as a scratch or insect bite, they can cause terrible problems—especially in any individual whose immune system is compromised.

Throughout the course of our evolution, our defensins have been protecting us by killing harmful bacteria. Much is known about defensins, including their structure, but they are extremely difficult and expensive to produce synthetically. Moreover, defensin molecules include components you would reject as foreign if they were produced by any body other than your own. This makes designing an off-the-shelf defensin-based drug a challenge.

So scientists set out to devise a stripped-down molecule made exclusively of elements that enable a defensin to attack a bacterium and that are found in everyone's defensins. They believed that the immune system would tolerate such a simplified molecule and that it would be much easier to manufacture and deliver to a patient.

There are, however, many different types of defensins and nearly unlimited ways of putting together simplified versions. Rather than go through the slow, expensive process of making and testing new defensins, researchers called on the power of computer-simulation technology to perform "in silico" experiments with a vast number of possible defensin molecules.

They found many promising molecules but, due to costs and regulatory impediments, tested only a few of them in people. These simplified defensin molecules killed bacteria on contact and behaved in other ways like their natural counterparts.

Unfortunately, the design of the original developers' clinical trials included flaws that triggered enough grief from regulators to drive the developers away from the project. However, others have picked up where they left off and are continuing the research.

As I indicated, this is only one of many new approaches to dealing with external biological threats to our health, and I find it significant that many of these breakthroughs look to our own biology for clues and solutions. This theme is appearing in many areas of scientific research, even in solar power, where the most promising new technologies are mimics of natural processes.

This modern, nature-based view of medicine will have its greatest impact in the most disruptive of all biotechnologies: anti-aging.

Chapter 31

"Off" Switches for Aging Accelerators

C hronic inflammation, dubbed "inflammaging" by gerontologist Claudio Franceschi, is an autoimmune disorder. In 2011, three scientists won the Nobel Prize in Medicine[47] for their work explaining how our immune system, which protects us when we're young, can attack us when we get older.

The immune response to injury and invasion is called the "inflammatory reflex." It's a complex mechanism responsible for healing salvageable cells and destroying and replacing those that can't be healed. It's essential to our health and survival but, ironically, the net benefit has dwindled with modern healthcare's success in keeping us alive for more years.

For most of human history, the most dangerous time in any person's life was infancy. Modern health care changed that, but during all of human existence, more people died from infection during infancy than from any other cause.

But not your grandparents. The fact that you're here now and reading this means that every one of your ancestors came out of the womb with an immune system on high, to deal with the myriad threats of the pre-modern eras.

Moreover, most of our grandmothers bore children at a much younger age than is common now. At a time when lives were far shorter, early marriage and childbirth were the rule rather than the exception. In the Middle Ages, the average age of *primigravida*, the first pregnancy, was sixteen or seventeen. Remember, that was the average; many women gave birth earlier. Accident and disease killed most people before they grew old, so the genes that favored maximum-drive immune systems were advantageous and were passed on to future generations.

---

47 http://www.nobelprize.org/nobel_prizes/medicine/laureates/2011/press.html

We've still got those genes, which means our immune systems are optimized for the short lifespans characteristic of past centuries. However, most people living today will reach old age (if they haven't gotten there already), and when they do, their immune systems will become trouble-makers.

Inflammaging

The always-on, pedal-to-the-metal immune systems that served human survival so well in pre-modern times and that continue to benefit young people become a liability as we age.

Autoimmune inflammation increases because our bodies seem to misinterpret the common ailments of aging as injury or invasion. This mistaken activation puts the immune system at cross purposes, trying to heal cells that have degraded through age while simultaneously trying to swap them out through apoptosis and replacement.

In most people, chronic inflammation increases year by year until it eventually triggers a life-ending cascade of negative effects. It's a vicious cycle that spins faster and faster until the organism itself fails.

Aging, we now know, is not linear. Like so many other things, it is a process that accelerates over time, and inflammaging is one of the most powerful drivers. It contributes to cancer, heart attack, lupus, irritable-bowel syndrome, macular degeneration, stroke, obesity, erectile dysfunction, allergies, psoriasis, Crohn's disease, endometriosis, rheumatoid arthritis, hair loss, and diseases of the thyroid, liver and other organs. I could go on.

This is why scientists have been searching for a way to control the auto-immune inflammation cycle. If we could stop chronic low-level inflammation, even cells damaged by past inflammation could heal. In animal studies, tissues seem to rejuvenate after inflammaging has been halted.

Inflammation is the primary accelerator of telomere loss, which is one reason so few of us reach our theoretical 120-year maximum life spans. Ending inflammaging won't restore lost telomeres, but it does slow their loss and thus extends life spans of animals.

In a body without chronic inflammation, aging would be more linear. It would happen, but it wouldn't accelerate. A substance that can stop the acceleration is the "holy grail" of drug research.

One of the most important projects of the 21st century is research into the immune system's alarm protein, NF-kB[48]. When we're young, the protein triggers a protective response to injury or infection that promptly turns itself off when it's no longer needed. But in older people, NF-kB never really shuts down, so the immune-system weapons it activates eventually turn against us.

One candidate for stopping age-related inflammation is *anatabine citrate*, a compound found in tobacco, eggplants, cauliflower and peppers. Until recently, it was sold over the counter as a nutraceutical. It has a remarkable safety record, supported by toxicity studies from Harvard.

Anatabine citrate increases neurotransmitter levels and was first used to help people stop smoking.[49] Unfortunately, the FDA viewed this natural product as a drug because in clinical trials it had succeeded in alleviating thyroiditis and type-2 diabetes. Because it works, the product was taken off the market.

I consider this a tragedy, but at this point, there's nothing I can do about it.

There aren't many stories this big in modern medicine. I recommend watching Dr. Fiona Crawford's presentation at the New College of Florida about the effects of anatabine citrate on traumatic brain injury.[50] This same data, as presented to a conference for neurologists, was cited by the FDA as a reason for pulling anatabine citrate from the over-the-counter market.

Aanatabine citrate is now in clinical trials outside the United States, so other scientists know that it's possible to safely turn off inflammaging without suppressing normal immune function. The compound likely will be approved in Europe or Japan within a few years. Then, after a few more years, it will become available again in the US, and I hope we're all still alive when it happens.

Because several hundred thousand Americans took the product when it was available, we know a lot about its effects. For many people suffering from arthritis and other inflammatory diseases (some of them life-threatening), the results were close to miraculous.

And there may be more to the benefits of controlling NF-kB than putting

---

48 Nuclear factor kappa B
49 Incidentally, nicotine on its own doesn't provide the "feel good" condition imparted by tobacco, which is why nicotine gum and patches do little to help anyone stop smoking.
50 See https://youtu.be/GmZRVxFXioA

a stop to inflammaging.

- Research from the Ohio State University Wexner Medical Center implicates over-activation of NF-kB as one of the ways cancers protect themselves from the immune system.
- The Albert Einstein College of Medicine in New York has published research showing that lowering the activation of NF-kB in the hypothalamus seems to slow aging. (The hypothalamus, located near the center of your head, is the master clock and hormone regulator of aging.)
- In animals, moderation of NF-kB in the hypothalamus alone led to significantly extended life spans and a prolonged youthful physical appearance.

Use of an NF-kB moderating compound would have an enormous impact, quickly reducing age-related diseases and extending health spans and life spans toward the 120-year mark. But we'll have to wait until the regulators give their permission.

Autophagy and Misfolded Proteins

Another line of research into premature aging is the role of autophagy. Autophagy means "self-eating." So why would we need to eat ourselves, and what does it have to do with aging?

Genes are natural nanomachines that synthesize the proteins that constitute and regulate our bodies. A gene operates by assembling a matching string of RNA, which in turn assembles a string of amino acids that folds itself into a specific protein. These strings are extremely long, and the folding process is complex. Imagine assembling a chain of simple components that you can rely on to fold itself into a functioning smartphone.

Occasionally, something goes wrong, and a protein folds incorrectly and won't function as it's supposed to. In some cases, misfolded proteins will damage the cell they're part of. In rare cases, they become prions, proteins that can transform other proteins into copies of themselves. That's how mad cow disease happens.

A young genome runs like a well-oiled machine. When the occasional transcription error yields a faulty (misfolded) protein, the defective goods are eliminated through autophagy and through the dissolving action of the acid-bearing lysosomes present in every cell.

As we age, however, protein-synthesis errors happen more frequently. At the same time, the autophagy-lysosome pathway is losing vigor, leaving misfolded proteins to accumulate and clog the works. Fortunately, it now seems possible to fix the problem by activating a biochemical switch in a cell's outer membrane called a sigma-1 receptor.

I was drawn into this topic when I learned of a sigma-1 receptor drug being tested on rodents that had gone blind from trauma-induced glaucoma. Turning numerous universally accepted truths upside down, the drug restored the rodents' sight. Seemingly dead optic nerves resumed functioning.

Since then, it's been found that activation of the sigma-1 receptor protects neurons, apparently by supporting autophagy. The enhanced autophagy cleans out the accumulated protein junk that's been clogging the neurons.

One of the most promising Alzheimer's drugs under development works by activating sigma-1 receptors. Alzheimer's involves a buildup of the misfolded protein amyloid beta, so it makes sense that turning on autophagy might help reverse the disease. Early trials on the drug indicate this is happening and that something else is going on. Acuity, or intelligence, in treated Alzheimer's mice instantly improves, long before autophagy could clear out the crystallized amyloids. Obviously, this was something of a surprise, but the even bigger surprise was that control mice without Alzheimer's also got smarter when given the drug.

It appears that the clutter of misfolded proteins in our brain cells acts like static, interfering with neural functioning and thought. Based on conversations with the researchers, I think we will have true sigma-1 receptor nootropics (smart drugs) in the near future. Since the regulatory agencies don't recognize "stupid" as a treatable disease, it will probably be approved as a prescription-only Alzheimer's preventative before it's made available directly to the public.

But this isn't the end of the story. Misfolded proteins are present in all cells and in higher concentrations as you age. Activating sigma-1 receptors should clear out the accumulated cellular debris that contributes to inflammation and to mitochondrial dysfunction. This is an extremely auspicious development for putting an end to premature aging.

Mitochondrial Dysfunction

Among the most exciting subjects of modern anti-aging research are mitochondria and the role of *nicotinamide adenine dinucleotide* (NAD) in their functioning.

As discussed earlier, mitochondria are tiny, bacteria-like organelles that reside in every cell. They have their own DNA, consisting of only 37 genes. They make up the biological power grid that uses food energy to produce adenosine triphosphate (ATP), the power-pack molecule that directly delivers the energy that drives every biochemical process.

ATP is uniquely important because it delivers the *only* energy a cell can use directly. If ATP production from your mitochondria is deficient, you have an energy crisis, no matter what you eat. There's evidence that deterioration of the ATP machinery causes the body to increase storage of food as fat, which contributes to obesity.

ATP is a molecular pistol. The adenosine handle has three phosphates attached as a kind of gun barrel. The two phosphates closest to the barrel are tightly bound. The third phosphate's bond, however, is looser. In the right conditions, the gun can be fired, releasing the third phosphate with its electrochemical energy. Molecular models of ATP such as the one below are even shaped somewhat like pistols.

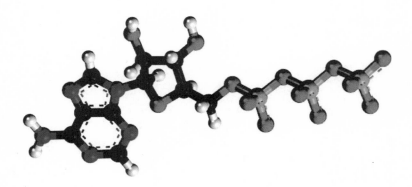

The energy released by the breaking of ATP's third phosphate bond directly powers innumerable biological processes. After the release, the mitochondrion burns glucose derived from food to reload the spent remains of the ATP molecule with a replacement third phosphate. This happens over and over, pretty much constantly.

You have quadrillions of mitochondria. Within a given cell, an army of them communicate with one another and with the cell's genome through the action of *nicotinamide adenine dinucleotide plus* (NAD$^+$). Unfortunately, as you age, NAD$^+$ becomes less abundant, and so the communication system degrades. The army deteriorates into a mob. Each mitochondrion is left to sputter on its own, isolated and on autopilot without the real-time information it needs to respond to changing cellular conditions. Without efficiently cooperating mitochondria, a fluttering energy supply stresses the cell.

The implications of what has been learned in recent years about mitochondria and age-related disease are enormous. A growing number of scientists—including more than a half-dozen Nobel Prize winners—believe that boosting NAD$^+$ levels will restore the efficient interaction of each mitochondrion with the rest of the cell... which could lead to significantly extended health spans.

A few years ago, the authors of *Mitochondrial Function as a Determinant of Life Span* proposed protecting mitochondrial function as a strategy for prolonging our lives. The paper described how mitochondrial function in muscle cells declines over time, suggesting that the decline may be related to lower oxygen uptake. This led the authors to recommend aerobic exercise as a solution.

While exercise does contribute to health, more recent research suggests other ways to prevent the decline of mitochondrial function, as discussed in the next chapter.

Chapter 32

Mitochondria—the Aliens Within

Mitochondria were discovered during the second half of the 19th century as improvements in microscopes and associated technology allowed closer examination of individual cells. What these cells within cells actually did, however, was unknown.

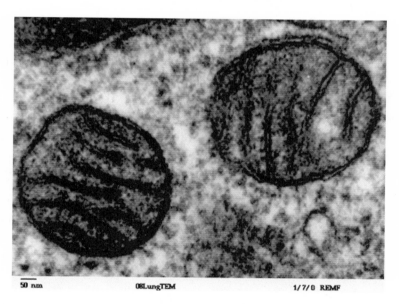

Transmission electron microscope image of a thin section cut through an area of mammalian lung tissue. The high magnification image shows mitochondria. (source: JEOL 100CX TEM Louisa Howard, Dartmouth)

Given the tininess of a mitochondrion and the primitive tools available for examining it, that's not surprising. A mitochondrion measures one micron

183

across—that's one thousandth of a millimeter. To put that in perspective, a human red blood cell is about five microns in size.

Textbook drawings typically show one or two mitochondria in a cell. In reality, some cells hold thousands, each drawing energy out of the chemical bonds of glucose to produce action-ready ATP molecules.

Your body holds about one-half pound of ATP, but that 8-ounce inventory turns over at an astounding rate. In just one day, you may go through an amount of ATP equal to your full body weight.

The Intelligent Grid

Mitochondria are radically different from all other organelles in a cell.

First, there's the matter of packaging. Every other large organelle, including the nucleus that protects the DNA, is contained within a membrane similar to the one that surrounds and encapsulates the entirety of the cell. Mitochondria are the only exception. A mitochondrion is surrounded by a double membrane layer, just like a bacterium.

Second, they're the only organelles with their own DNA. And whereas the DNA of your genome is linear (with two ends), mitochondrial DNA is circular, with no ends at all, just like bacterial DNA.

This similarity of mitochondria to bacteria is extremely important. Bacteria are independent organisms, but they can cooperate in astonishing ways by transferring chemically coded information among themselves. This helps them, for example, to pass immunity to antibiotics to others of their species.

Scientists have harnessed the power of circular DNA to build a bacterial computer capable of solving complex problems. This is not merely some interesting trivia or an exhibition of virtuosity. It underscores that our mitochondria function like a biological computer network.

A single mitochondrion has 37 genes, including 14 distinct protein-coding genes, which seems a tiny endowment compared with the 25,000 protein-coding genes of your chromosomes. Each mitochondrion, however, carries multiple copies of its circular DNA, and there can be thousands of mitochondria in a cell. A network that complex and will perform badly without communication and coordination among all the elements.

Healthy mitochondria, like bacteria, frequently divide and frequently merge with other mitochondria. However, they lack the repair capabilities of a bacterium. Repair is controlled through the genome in the cell's nucleus, which oversees the mitochondrial network. That's one reason a breakdown in communication between mitochondria and the genome is so harmful.

We don't yet understand everything mitochondria do, but it's known that only a small portion of mitochondrial DNA is involved with the production of ATP. This leaves a lot of computational capacity for other functions. Scientists are beginning to view this intelligent grid in a new light. More importantly, we're gaining a better understanding of how the network deteriorates as we age and how the deterioration damages our health.

The big anti-aging news, however, is that there are ways to restore the network, even when we are quite old.

When the Lines of Communication Break Down, So Do We

A mitochondrion's activity needs to adjust as the energy needs of its cell fluctuate, and for that to happen, all of a cell's mitochondria need to communicate with the genome. In a healthy cell, proteins made in the genome travel to the mitochondria and announce the cell's current ATP needs. Many scientists now believe that NAD^+ is the main messenger. However NAD^+ levels fall with age, leaving the communication pathways of metabolic regulation to gradually go bad.

One way to increase NAD^+ levels is to ingest NAD precursors, molecules that the body will metabolize into NAD^+. A Harvard study by Sinclair *et al.* found pronounced improvement in the muscle cells of mice that had been injected with an NAD^+ precursor.[51]

A 2013 Harvard Medical School article reports, "Examining muscle from two-year-old mice that had been given the NAD-producing compound for just one week, the researchers looked for indicators of insulin resistance, inflammation, and muscle wasting. In all three instances, tissue from the mice resembled that of six-month-old mice. In human years, this would be like a 60-year-old converting to a 20-year-old in these specific areas."[52]

---

51 David Andrew Sinclair, Harvard geneticist and aging researcher, is best known for research into resveratrol.
52 See https://hms.harvard.edu/news/genetics/new-reversible-cause-aging-12-19-13

How could this be? How could NAD$^+$ precursors reverse the effect of aging?

Allow me to speculate. Initially the rate is very low, but from the time you are born, if not before, it happens every day: the DNA in some of your mitochondria is mutated through the action of free radicals, natural radiation, or other interference. The mutations accumulate and eventually impair mitochondrial function.

It's no surprise that mitochondrial DNA is fragile. With only 37 genes, mitochondrial DNA is too simple and too spare to repair itself. Lacking the sophisticated maintenance mechanisms of the nuclear genome, your mitochondria if left to themselves are doomed to fail and destined to take you with them.

There is, however, another possibility: restore the ability of mitochondria to communicate. That reboots the genome's mitochondrial repair function. The nuclear genome then directs the cell to favor replication of the healthiest mitochondrial DNA and to abandon the rest. This rejuvenates the cellular energy grid and thereby the cells themselves.

NAD$^+$ Precursors

Supplementing the cell's supply of the molecules needed for NAD$^+$ production raises NAD$^+$ levels in humans and animals. The benefits have been measured over short periods of time... though I would expect the real benefits to be more long term and hence more difficult to measure accurately without extended studies.

Some NAD$^+$ precursors are "naturally occurring," meaning they are already found in our cells, which allows the material to be sold over the counter

Nicotinamide Riboside

One naturally occurring NAD$^+$ precursor is *nicotinamide riboside* (NR), which has been studied in clinical trials by Dr. Charles Brenner at the University of Iowa.

So does NR increase NAD$^+$ levels in humans?

It does, and even better, it seems to be completely safe.

Does this make it one of the anti-aging breakthroughs we've been waiting for?

It's hard to get past "Maybe," for several reasons. In the thinking of the FDA, testing any compound for specific diseases in human trials makes the compound a "drug." So a human trial of NR for a mitochondrial disease would invite the FDA to bump NR from the shelves of the supplement market.

Human longevity studies could prove NR's value for life extension, but you don't really know how something affects a life span until you've waited long enough for test subjects to die. So a valid controlled study would take decades and thousands of people.

However, some scientists believe we already know enough to warrant use of NR for life extension. MIT biologist Leonard Guarente is best known for his research into the sirtuin genes, which are activated via calorie restriction. This article[53] about Elysium Health and Guarente's decisions to formulate a nutraceutical product line featuring NR got a lot of attention.

Guarente also included pterostilbene in his product, a phytochemical from blueberries known to activate the sirtuins. Apparently, he expects a synergistic effect of the sirtuin activators with NR.

"NAD replacement is one of the most exciting things happening in the biology of aging," says Nir Barzilai, director of the Institute for Aging Research at the Albert Einstein College of Medicine in New York, who has coauthored scientific papers with Guarente but is not involved in his company. "The frustration in our field is that we have shown we can target aging, but the FDA does not [recognize it] as an indication."

Even skeptics quoted in the article are only partly skeptical.

"There is enough evidence to be excited, but not completely compelling evidence," said Brian K. Kennedy, CEO of the California-based Buck Institute for Research on Aging.

I'm about the same age as Guarente, so I may not have time for "completely compelling evidence." I take both of the compounds in his product.

---

53 http://www.technologyreview.com/news/534636/the-anti-aging-pill/

Oxaloacetate

Another NAD$^+$ precursor I've taken for several years is a variant of oxaloacetate (OAA), a molecule that occurs naturally in a mitochondrion's production of ATP and in other cellular functions.

Adding oxaloacetate to the diets of animals extends their lives, but for many years the point was academic, because the compound quickly decomposes unless it is stored at a very low temperature. Then, in 2006, an engineer struck by oxaloacetate's anti-aging benefits produced a variant that is stable at room temperature, which opened the door for supplementation.

A patent on the process of stabilizing oxaloacetate was granted in 2015. The University of Kansas Medical Center Research Institute has completed preliminary trials for using the substance to treat Alzheimer's disease and Parkinson's disease. Happily, the product, named benaGene, is still available through a private company, Terra Biological LLC.

Oxaloacetate increases the availability of NAD$^+$ through an entirely different mechanism than NR. This suggests that the two compounds may be complementary. So I take both.

Animal studies have shown that a third compound, acetyl-L-carnitine, works synergistically with oxaloacetate, so I take it as well. Acetyl-L-carnitine is a naturally occurring substance that breaks down in the blood to transport fatty acids into the mitochondria for conversion to ATP.

One important study showed that rats suffering from induced stroke regained their ability to learn when treated with oxaloacetate and acetyl-L-carnitine. This seems like a very good sign, since in humans the ability to form memories tends to decrease with age. Given the option, I'd like to preserve the ability to learn as long as possible. Maybe, someday, I'll even learn how to spell "rhythm" without a spell checker and remember my in-laws' names. Many users of either NR or oxaloacetate report a lifting of mental "fogginess."

There has been a lot of research on oxaloacetate, but a paper published in the *Journal of Human Molecular Genetics* stands out.[54] Its reports that oxaloacetate increases energy production in the brain, improves processing of insulin for greater energy and resistance to type-2 diabetes, reduces

---

54 See http://hmg.oxfordjournals.org/content/23/24/6528 Oxford Journals
Medicine & Health & Science & Mathematics
Human Molecular Genetics

inflammation in the body, and stimulates neuron growth in mice.

Yes, there have been drugs that work in mice but not in people. However, mitochondrial processes are similar across mammalian species, so it's likely that anything that helps mitochondria in mice will help mitochondria in you... and in your dog, too.

Another supplement for ATP energy production is ubiquinol, a form of coenzyme Q10 (CoQ10) that appears to be especially active. Ubiquinol is part of the electron transport chain for synthesizing ATP. It's available in most stores that sell supplements, as is acetyl-L-carnitine.

Each compound increases NAD^+ via a different pathway, so they might complement one another. In time, clinical trials will nail down the most beneficial combination and dosages of NAD^+ precursors. Until then, we're only guessing, but, as Dr. Guarente suggests, I'm too old to wait for perfect information.

Chapter 33

Erasing the Scars of Aging

Many effects of aging can't be detected directly, but some are obvious, such as wrinkles and impaired flexibility. *Flexibility* is the relevant word here. When skin loses its flexibility, it wrinkles and sags. When tissues that connect the arms, legs and other limbs to the rest of the body lose flexibility, movement becomes slower and more constrained.

Inflexibility that goes unseen is an even more serious problem. Half of all organ failures involve fibrosis, the growth of inflexible scar tissue. Two systemic—and frequently fatal—fibrotic disorders are liver disease and pulmonary fibrosis. Fibrosis can also cause blindness, kidney disease, and arthritis.

Most of us think of this scarring of our bodies as inevitable. It isn't.

Recall from Chapter 28 that as a strategy for fooling the immune system, tumors build structures out galectin-3s that resemble scar tissue. Supplementing conventional chemotherapy with a plant sugar that blocks galectin-3 interfered with that tumor survival strategy, opened tumors to attack, and restored the organs of mice to a youthful, non-fibrotic condition.

Even apart from its importance in treating cancer, this astonishing discovery is one of the greatest anti-aging breakthroughs of our era, but almost no one seems to appreciate the implications. Blocking galextin-3s with a certain plant sugar improved organ health throughout the body by decreasing fibrosis. Adding to the picture are animal studies showing that when the galectin-3 gene is deactivated, fibrosis can't happen at all.

Fibrotic tissues, like most tissues, renew themselves continuously with new cells. So if galectin-3 activity is reduced, we can expect fibrotic materials to fade and make room for healthy cells. In other words, blocking galectin-3 won't just prevent fibrosis, it will reverse it.

While fibrosis is a healthy function (when there is a need for building scar tissue), it's one of the many mechanisms that get out of whack as we age, further accelerating the aging process. An effective and safe anti-fibrotic would therefore be a powerful anti-aging therapy. Though research in this area is much further along than most people know, there's still much to explore. However, I'm convinced that galectin-3 blocking therapies will reverse the loss of flexibility associated with old age, thereby increasing the quality of life and total life spans.

GDF11 and Vampire Therapy

I'm proud of an obscure reference to myself in Robert Heinlein's book *To Sail Beyond the Sunset*. It came from something I said to him in his home in Bonny Doon, California. I was there because Heinlein had asked me to write an article for the *Wall Street Journal* about him and his forthcoming book, *The Cat Who Walks Through Walls*.

So I chose the wine, and his wife Ginny cooked several meals that day as the conversation extended into the morning hours. Pixel, the cat that inspired the book's title, was there as well. Just as he did in the book, the cat seemed to appear and disappear at will. If you're interested, the article is still online at the Heinlein Society website.[55]

The Cat Who Walks Through Walls is interesting to Heinlein fans for several reasons. One is that it may be read as a sequel to Heinlein's *The Moon Is a Harsh Mistress*, though it also continues story lines found in *The Number of the Beast*. One of the main characters is Lazarus Long, who first appeared in *Methuselah's Children*, a story involving people who are extremely long-lived.

Heinlein gave two explanations for his characters' longevity. One was selective breeding, which we now know is entirely plausible. I foresee dating sites soon to come where people with the super-ager CETP gene can find one another. The other mechanism for extending life spans was periodic transfusions from very young donors, so-called "vampire therapy."

Of course, we're talking about science fiction here; nobody really believed young blood could extend lives. If they had, the hypothesis would have been easy to test. In fact, 73 years after *Methuselah's Children* was

---

55 http://www.heinleinsociety.org/rah/conservativeview.html

serialized in *Astounding Science Fiction*, such an experiment was performed at the Stanford University School of Medicine using mice.

Interestingly, the senior author of the Stanford blood study, Tony Wyss-Coray, Ph.D., noted that the experiment could have been done 20 years earlier. I think it could have been done long before that. The procedure was simple: Eight times over a period of 24 days, the team gave 18-month-old mice blood plasma (blood from which all cells have been removed) from 3-month-old mice. When the aged mice underwent a rodent IQ test, they showed significant improvements.

The overview of the study, published in the journal Nature, states:

> As human lifespan increases, a greater fraction of the population is suffering from age-related cognitive impairments, making it important to elucidate a means to combat the effects of aging. Here we report that exposure of an aged animal to young blood can counteract and reverse pre-existing effects of brain aging at the molecular, structural, functional and cognitive level. Genome-wide microarray analysis of heterochronic parabionts—in which circulatory systems of young and aged animals are connected—identified synaptic plasticity–related transcriptional changes in the hippocampus of aged mice.

In other words, the brains of the older mice given transfusions from the young mice didn't simply perform better — they showed physical signs of rejuvenation. Clearly, this is a pretty big deal. To reiterate, the last sentence of the summary says, "Our data indicate that exposure of aged mice to young blood late in life is capable of rejuvenating synaptic plasticity and improving cognitive function."

Many of the reports about the Stanford study focused on the possibility of isolating the rejuvenating factors in young blood and using them on their own. A prime candidate is the protein expressed by the growth differentiation factor 11 (GDF11) gene. GDF11 protein production decreases with age; prior research showed that it has rejuvenating effects in parts of the body other than the brain.

Heinlein's common sense continues to impress, but it's unlikely we would need to use blood itself to exploit his idea. (There are, by the way, stories of "vampire therapy" being offered in certain very high-end clinics outside the United States. You can probably guess where.)

Several experiments have demonstrated[56] that age-related damage to the heart muscle in older mice can also be reversed by GDF11 proteins from younger animals. This is of enormous interest to researchers, because heart muscle cells generally don't regenerate in older mammals, human or otherwise. As it stands today, heart attack damage is permanent damage, and it increases the odds of another heart attack.

I'm baffled that US healthcare agencies haven't made GDF11 therapy a priority, given the sky-high costs of heart disease. Regardless, I think it will be available in the near future, perhaps outside the US.

I don't believe, however, that the therapy will involve injections of GDF11 itself. An exogenous dose of a bioactive protein, even if it's naturally occurring, tends to upset the regulatory axis that balances all the complex processes running in the body. Side effects wouldn't just be possible, they'd be likely.

Fortunately, there are better ways to restore GDF11 to youthful levels—including stem cell implants and DNA vaccines. We know from the experience of people who take growth hormone releasing hormone (GHRH), which I will discuss next, that hormones produced in the body are recognized and integrated into the entire system of hormonal regulation. This means there may be very few if any negative side effects. Several scientists I communicate with regularly believe their firms could deliver this therapy at moderate cost (assuming regulatory approval).

Growth Hormone Releasing Hormone

A few years ago, human growth hormone (hGH) was the hottest topic in life extension. Users saw remarkable benefits, including fat loss, restoration of hair and skin, and increased muscle mass. Too much growth hormone, however, can cause a variety of unpleasant side effects, including joint swelling and pain, carpal tunnel syndrome, and an increased risk of diabetes. In severe cases, acromegaly (thickening of the bones of the jaw, fingers, and toes) may take place.

A precursor, growth hormone releasing hormone (GHRH), yields the same benefits as hGH but with fewer problems. Its action to raise levels of

---

56 http://www.nature.com/cr/journal/v24/n12/full/cr2014107a.html

hGH is subject to the body's mechanisms for limiting hGH to safe levels and for maintaining a balance with other hormones, sparing the user most if not all of the unwanted side effects.

Then why don't more people use GHRH? Practicality. It's difficult to manufacture and hence is ridiculously expensive. Moreover, its half-life in the body is short, so an effective therapy would require multiple injections per day. And given the regulatory bias against anti-aging therapies, only someone with a condition involving grave hGH deficiency, such as AIDS, could legally get access to GHRH therapy.

In the agricultural world, however, things are different. A DNA vaccine that triggers natural GHRH production has been given to tens of thousands of farm animals in Australia and South Korea. The vaccinated animals are not only stronger, leaner, more fertile, less prone to disease, and smarter than their untreated counterparts, they significantly outlive them. One of my greatest frustrations is that even though this biotechnology could be adapted for humans with little investment or research, regulatory barriers prevent it. That's why you're not getting the health and longevity benefits now being enjoyed by thousands of sheep. Nonetheless, I'm convinced this technology will reach the human market in the near future.

Another strategy for boosting GHRH is to engraft GHRH-producing stem cells, perhaps in conjunction with BAT cells, which you'll read about in the next chapter.

Chapter 34

BAT Science: The Dark Fat Returns

School children learn about their most vital organs. They're taught they wouldn't be able to live without the heart, the stomach, the intestines, the lungs, or the brain that controls them all. They learn about the liver and kidneys and that the skin itself is also an organ.

The science you learned as a child, however, is not settled. The current revolution in biological knowledge has brought truly exciting discoveries about an organ you've probably never heard of.

I'm talking about fat.

If the categorization of skin as an organ seems strange, then thinking of fat as an organ is even stranger. A large portion of the American population is fighting obesity, which may be the single most damaging accelerator of aging. Americans seldom go for more than a few hours without eating. As a result, many take in food energy faster than they burn it, i.e., they gain weight.

In recent years, the US government's decades-long effort to promote the consumption of carbohydrates instead of dietary fats has slowly been discredited. While this is clearly a good thing, it's not where the real action regarding obesity is. In my opinion, the most important discovery is about a certain type of fat that calibrates our metabolisms and matches calorie burning with calorie intake.

Most of the fat in your body is *white fat* (white adipose tissue, or WAT), which stores excess nutrition. While WAT is the conspicuous culprit in weight gain, its build-up appears related to changes in the *brown fat* (brown adipose tissue, or BAT) that makes up a small fraction of total body fat. Researchers have discovered that BAT is a vital organ—in fact, the age-related loss of brown fat may lead to gains in white fat, in obesity and in the maladies those increases bring on.

These two tissues differ in important ways. A white fat cell holds a huge droplet of lipids, leaving little room for other cell organelles such as the mitochondria needed for burning food energy. A brown fat cell, as the other part of this fatty yin and yang, contains just a few small droplets of lipids but numerous mitochondria whose sole purpose is to burn calories. If white fat cells are our body's firewood stockpile, then brown fat cells are the stoves. To burn calories, all that's needed is to turn the brown fat cells on.

Not long ago, scientists thought of BAT only in connection with animal hibernation, naming it the "hibernating gland." Their focus has only recently shifted to the role that BAT loss plays in age-related obesity.

According to the journal *Adipocyte*, "it has been estimated that as little as 50 g of BAT (less than 0.1% of body weight) could utilize up to 20% of basal caloric needs if maximally stimulated. This energy-expending role makes BAT an important potential tool for combating the complications of human obesity."

To translate, stimulating your seven tablespoons of brown fat (which is normally found in the upper back and chest around the scapula and clavicle) could increase your calorie burn rate by 20%—even while you sit perfectly still. We used to believe that BAT is activated primarily by cool temperatures. Recent research indicates that it is also turned on when children consume more calories than they need. The good news is that the BAT furnace is so good at producing heat, you don't actually feel cold when it's turned on. It also activates to rid the body of unneeded calories. If regularly activated, BAT burns so many calories that becoming or staying obese is nearly impossible. Eat a donut, burn a donut.

Sounds good, but we tend to lose brown fat as we age. If you have children, you've undoubtedly seen BAT thermogenesis in action. Small children seem impervious to low temperatures that have their parents bundled up and shivering. When my kids were toddlers and slept in diapers, they routinely kicked off their covers at night, even when temperatures dropped to the low sixties. If you touched them, they seemed to radiate heat.

One theory is that BAT atrophies from disuse. Thanks to indoor heating and modern cold-weather clothing, few of us get the exposure to cold that's needed to activate brown adipose tissue. Another theory is that a nutrient missing from modern diets may be responsible for the loss of BAT. It's also possible that, like our thymus glands, BAT simply shrinks with age.

The decrease in brown fat typically correlates with, or perhaps causes, an increase in white fat.

By reducing fat stores, the increased caloric burn rate would indirectly influence many metabolic and cardiovascular issues, but it seems that the role of BAT in these processes is much more direct than that.

An article published in the *Journal of Clinical Investigation* entitled, "Brown Adipose Tissue Regulates Glucose Homeostasis And Insulin Sensitivity," states that BAT has a direct effect on molecules involved in diabetes. When brown fat cells were transplanted to a mouse that lacked them, the results were dramatic: "By 8–12 weeks following transplantation, recipient mice had improved glucose tolerance, increased insulin sensitivity, lower body weight, decreased fat mass, and a complete reversal of high-fat diet-induced insulin resistance."

Triglycerides are the fatty acids our white fat cells hoard and the fuel our brown fat cells burn. BAT also disposes of glucose and produces adipokines, important signaling molecules for controlling inflammatory and metabolic processes.

All this new evidence about the organ we didn't know we had (but very much need) makes the news that we lose it with age hard to take. But regenerative medicine has the power to restore BAT with an excitingly simple procedure that has been done numerous times in animals.

Though it may sound like science-fiction, it is now possible to make tanker trucks full of purified BAT cells. The next step would be to implant the cells in their normal location, around the scapula, a procedure similar to cosmetic or reconstructive surgeries commonly carried out today.

But how could this solution be made permanent?

Reconstructive and cosmetic surgery draw unwanted fat from the belly, thighs or glutes and inject it elsewhere to fill in a scar or wrinkle. It works, for a while, but in time the relocated cells drift away, because conventional surgery does nothing to anchor the transplanted cells in their new neighborhood. Cell drift assures that the effects of the surgery, however welcome, are transitory.

Cells that have developed naturally are anchored by an extracellular matrix (ECM), which is a scaffolding or structural framework made of water, proteins, and complex carbohydrates such as collagen. An ECM not only separates cells, it keeps them in place and performs functions specific to the type of cells it contains.

The problem of cell drift has recently been solved, however, and the solution is on the road to regulatory approval. ECMs have been created using materials that exist naturally in the body that can be modified to fit the needs of specific cell types. These ECMs can be made rigid enough to allow growth of connective tissue in the joints or pliable enough to allow the use of a patient's own fat cells for breast reconstruction. Most importantly, these revolutionary ECMs are replaced over time by the patient's own natural ECM, giving permanence to cell transplants.

The discovery of BAT's benefits will help end the epidemic of metabolic syndrome that contributes to most of the biggest medical problems, including type-2 diabetes, Alzheimer's disease, heart disease, and cancer. It's exciting to find that we can actually do something to restore BAT—not only to slim our waists and feel better, but to extend our lifespans and lower healthcare costs.

Right now, a suite of transformative sciences are emerging that complement each other wonderfully. We don't yet understand which, if any, of the aging accelerators are preeminent. Inflammation, fibrosis, mitochondrial dysfunction, protein misfolding, and loss of BAT may all be separate failures —or they may be linked by a master cause.

One thing is clear, though: blocking any of these degenerators would extend health spans and solve the financial crisis brought on by the aging of society.

Chapter 35

Regenerative Medicine:
The Game Changer

Regenerative stem cell medicine may be the most disruptive biotechnology in history. It could do more than just slow aging and delay the onset of disease. It could reverse cellular aging and restore youthful health to older cells, to organs and to whole organisms... including human beings.

Among the anti-aging therapies, stem cell medicine is unique. Up to this point, I've covered strategies to extend health spans toward our maximum natural life span of about 120 years. With those strategies, you'd maintain good health until you reached your Hayflick Limit and your cells ran out of telomeres. Then, and only then, you would die.

Regenerative medicine, however, *overcomes* the Hayflick Limit by restoring youthful telomere strands. As each cell in your body wore out, it would be replaced with a younger cell with a full set of telomeres.

No fetuses need to be troubled to advance this science. The noisy controversy about capturing embryonic stem cells (eSCs) for use in research has become a sterile debate, thanks to the availability of induced Pluripotent Stem cells (iPS) through the technology explained below.

iPS—the Immortal Cells

One of the most exciting developments in modern medicine is the production of induced pluripotent stem cells (iPS), which for all practical purposes are identical to embryonic stem cells. They are rejuvenated completely, they replicate indefinitely, and they can be differentiated into any cell type.

Like embryonic stem cells, iPS cells are immortal in the sense that they have the "immortalizing" telomerase gene switched on, making them essentially zero years old until they are engineered to become adult cells with full sets of telomeres.

As it happens, I've had skin cells taken from inside my left arm and transformed into iPS cells. Here is a picture.

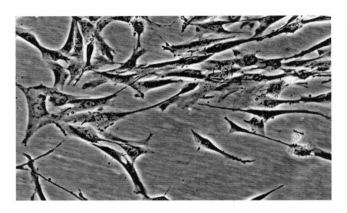

Some of those cells were later put through a process to restore their early embryonic condition, with the telomerase gene switched on. That made them identical to the embryonic stem cells I came from. Because they have my DNA, they can be returned to my body with no risk of immune rejection (a big advantage over cells derived from eSC lines).

The next picture is a clump of those immortalized pluripotent stem cells.

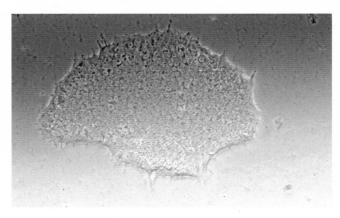

The immortalized cells could be turned into healthy, youthful replacement cells of any type—for example endothelial precursor stem cells, which replace the lining of the cardiovascular systems. Or they could be engineered to become cartilage or other connective tissues to replace joints and tendons. Anything my body might need.I chose to have my iPS cells engineered to become youthful heart muscle cells (cardiomyocytes) because anyone will appreciate what they are. Creating those heart muscle cells began by activating the appropriate genes in a few of the iPS cells. Then the transformed cells were multiplied to yield a pure population of identical cells.[57]

Here's a video—https://youtu.be/xd8HmNFPUeU. The engineered cells self-assemble and begin to beat regularly, just like my heart. We don't have regulatory approval to inject these cells back into me, but based on animal experiments, there is little doubt that they could replace older, less functional heart muscle cells and repair any damage my heart might suffer.

If I had a choice of stem cell therapies, however, I would choose to have my iPS cells engineered to become endothelial precursors. These are the stem cells residing in the marrow of your large bones that differentiate to become the cells of your immune system and of your endothelium, which is the thin layer of cells that line the inside of your cardiovascular system, including your heart and the tiniest capillaries in the back of your eyes.

There is a saying among gerontologists that you're as old as your endothelium. When you're young, these barrier cells perform a multitude of functions that keep your body robust and healthy. The endothelium, however, does not repair itself on site. Instead, the endothelial precursors in the bone marrow enter the blood system and circulate, checking for failing endothelial cells along the way and replacing any that are found.

A youthful endothelium is a wonderful thing. Perfectly smooth, it won't allow the buildup of the plaques of atherosclerosis. It's involved in the growth of new blood vessels for wound healing and organ repair as well as clotting, and it produces nitric oxide, the gaseous and most important neurotransmitter in the body.

Nitric oxide is the trigger for vasodilation, the widening of blood vessels that allows increased blood circulation when needed. As the endothelium

---

57 Using iPS cells has another big advantage over using eSC cells. Producing cell types from eSCs involves letting the cells develop and then trying to separate only the desired type from the mix. The separating is impossible to do perfectly, so transplanting the cells into the body can result in tumor-like growths that occur when a cell lodges at the wrong location.

ages and nitric oxide production falls, blood flow fails to rise when needed and the result is hypertension, or high blood pressure. Hypertension in turn causes heart disease, stroke, arterial disease, kidney failure, retinopathy, erectile dysfunction, and macular degeneration.

Animal tests have shown remarkable results from endothelial stem cell therapy. Researchers used a drug to destroy the bone marrow of aged cows. Then rejuvenated endothelial precursors were injected into the animals and also into a control group whose bone marrow had not been disturbed.

Following the procedure, there was no difference between the condition of the control group and of the cows whose bone marrow had been destroyed. In both groups, the rejuvenated endothelial precursors migrated to the bone marrow. This is important because it wasn't just cows lacking bone marrow or endothelial precursors that accepted the replacements. Cows with intact bone marrow also accepted the superior, younger replacements.

There is genius built into our DNA. Our bodies can recognize superior materials, so the aged stem cells were jettisoned in favor of the younger versions. Natural biological systems recognize the superiority of rejuvenated cells and spontaneously incorporate them in replacement for old and damaged cells.

Equipped with new endothelial precursor stem cells, both groups of cows experienced a gradual rejuvenation of their cardiovascular systems. If this procedure were performed in humans, delivering a youthful cardiovascular system without surgery, the cost would be less than $20,000. Even at five times that amount, the cost would still be far less than paying for heart bypass surgery or for a stroke caused by a failing endothelium.

The potential applications of regenerative medicine are nearly unlimited. Because stem cells come equipped with self-assembly instructions, they largely know what to do, and they do it. In experiments for the replacement of retinal cells to cure blindness, stem cells injected in a major artery found their way to the back of the eyes. Delivery techniques are going to be far more targeted than that, but the point is that the self-assembling abilities of stem cells make these therapies much easier than we imagined.

Other scientists are working on regenerative stem cell therapy for joint and connective tissue repair as well as liver and kidney disease.

Until recently, I wasn't particularly optimistic about the timeline for regenerative medicine, but deregulation in Japan is changing everything. Today it's possible to test the safety of a stem cell procedure in Japan and offer a therapy within six months. When people with failing hearts and clogged arteries begin to report the effects of a nonsurgical therapy that rejuvenates the cardiovascular system, the demand for this technology will be unstoppable. The FDA will get trampled.

Chapter 36

The Real Convergence

As baby boomers grow older, they will demand therapies to slow the effects of aging. They won't take "no" for an answer, even if getting "yes" requires travel to the Cayman Islands, Japan, or other jurisdictions with a free market for health care.

The pressure from the aging of society is going to force our healthcare system to shift to delaying or preventing the age-related conditions that lead to cancer, heart disease, dementia, arthritis, and other maladies— even though the transformation won't be convenient for most established healthcare companies. At the moment, though, the budget for anti-aging research is less than one percent of the money being spent to find treatments for disease. This will change.

We've already seen remarkable advances in anti-aging medicine despite the low levels of funding. It's not that we've solved all the problems; in fact, we don't yet know all the factors that contribute to aging. Still, the progress that has been made is stunning.

Anti-aging therapies and regenerative medicine are only part of the solution, however. In the world of technology, people have for decades used the word "convergence" to describe the coming-together of various electronic devices. The real convergence, however, is the coming-together of healthcare, mobile devices, robotics, artificial intelligence, and genomics.

The number of people who are having their genomes mapped is skyrocketing as the cost plummets. More importantly, an increasing number of those genome maps are being linked to medical records, giving bioinformaticians extraordinary insight into the genetic causes of disease. As this continues, more and more information will emerge on the consequences of lifestyle and supplement use.

The diagnostic power of artificial intelligence will grow. Your genome map and your medical experience will be cross-correlated with information from millions of other individuals. Your mobile device will send real-time information to a shared data system that will respond with personalized health advice. The final step in the convergence will come when your iPS cells are stored in an automated laboratory where personalized cell therapies will be prepared robotically.

At least one company, the leader in stem cell therapeutics, has already started working with a medical robotics company to automate the conversion of adult cells into iPS cells and then into specific cell types as needed. The diagnostic tools in your mobile device will tell the system to begin making cellular replacements that will be ready the moment you need them.

We live in fascinating times. For most of my life, we regular folk have been lectured about the horrors of overpopulation and the need to reduce birth rates. Those of us who actually understood the demographic trends knew the overpopulation story was nonsense, but it's hard to fight fearmongering with arithmetic.

As a result, I and other "overpopulation deniers" spent a lot of time being both annoyed and discouraged: annoyed that individuals who claim the mantle of science were spouting malarkey, and discouraged because so many supposedly educated people believed them. Finally, we're seeing the fixation on overpopulation begin to fade.

Edmund Burke was right when he pointed out that our species can learn, but only from experience. As the old paradigms break down, new technologies will be adopted more rapidly. And whether I live to see it or not, we are looking at a bright new world indeed.

Afterword: Final Thoughts

Scientific discovery, especially in the arena of biotechnology, has accelerated to a mind-boggling pace in just the last decade. More progress is now being made in the space of weeks than was made in most years of the 20th century. While the speed of scientific discovery is powering solutions to our most critical problems and ushering in an era of almost unimaginably widespread wealth and health, it also makes the archaic technology of information-sharing called "the book" obsolete for publicizing the current state of biotechnology.

In the short time that the manuscript I wrote was being turned into a book, there have been major biological discoveries that are even more exciting than what you have just read about. The text in your hands reflects a state of knowledge that is already becoming outdated.

Science-fiction writer Neal Stephenson envisioned a new book technology that constantly updates, a vision now possible with the internet. Douglas Adams presented a similar vision in his *Hitchiker's Guide to the Galaxy*.

For the nonce, I'll rely on my weekly and monthly newsletters to cure the constant obsolescing of the picture of state of the biological sciences. You can register for a complimentary subscription to the weekly publication here: http://www.mauldineconomics.com/tech

Notes

Books

Thompson, Warren Simpson. *Population Problems*. New York, London, McGraw-Hill Book Co., 1942.

Steven Pinker. *The Blank Slate*. New York, 2002. http://stevenpinker.com/publications/blank-slate

Freeman Dyson. *Dreams of Earth and Sky*. New York, 2015. http://www.amazon.com/Dreams-Earth-Sky-Freeman-Dyson/dp/1590178548

Michael West. *The Immortal Cell: One Scientist's Quest to Solve the Mystery of Human Aging*. Doubleday, 2003. https://books.google.com/books/about/The_Immortal_Cell.html?id=SZnuAAAAMAAJ

Eric Davidson. *The Regulatory Genome: Gene Regulatory Networks in Development And Evolution*. 2006. http://www.sciencedirect.com/science/book/9780120885633

George M. Church, Ed Regis. *Regenesis: How Synthetic Biology Will Reinvent Nature and Ourselves*. 2012. http://www.amazon.com/Regenesis-Synthetic-Biology-Reinvent-Ourselves/dp/0465075703

Joseph Schumpeter. *Capitalism, Socialism, and Democracy*. United States 1942. https://read.amazon.com/kp/embed?asin=B000SEPDJ6&reshareId=032ZGQWFHCZ704TQZWNX&reshareChannel=system

211

Joseph Schumpeter. *Business Cycles: A Theoretical, Historical and Statistical Analysis of the Capitalist Process.* http://www.amazon.com/Business-Cycles-Theoretical-Historical-Statistical/dp/1578985560

Gary Becker. *Human Capital.* The University of Chicago Press, 1993. http://www.press.uchicago.edu/ucp/books/book/chicago/H/bo3684031.html

Papers: Demography

National Institute on Aging (NIA), World Health Organization. *Global Health and Aging.* NIH Publication no. 11-7737, October 2011. https://d2cauhfh6h4x0p.cloudfront.net/s3fs-public/global_health_and_aging.pdf?q.52VK49USX58EJwZ3BjLl.yphsH2T_h

Arias, Elizabeth. *United States Life Tables,* 2003, revised March 28, 2007. CDC, National Center for Health Statistics. http://www.cdc.gov/nchs/data/nvsr/nvsr54/nvsr54_14.pdf

National Institute on Aging, Institute for Social Research at the University of Michigan. *Growing Older in America: The Health & Retirement Study.* University of Michigan, Institute for Social Research, 2016. http://hrsonline.isr.umich.edu/index.php?p=dbook

Abraham, Katharine G. and Harris, Benjamin H. *Better Financial Security in Retirement? Realizing the Promise of Longevity Annuities.* Brookings Institute 2014; revised February 2015. http://www.brookings.edu/~/media/images/abraham_harris_paper_rev4.pdf

The Canadian Institute for Health Information. *National Health Expenditure Trends, 1975 to 2015.* CIHA 2015. https://www.cihi.ca/sites/default/files/document/nhex_trends_narrative_report_2015_en.pdf

National Institute on Aging. *Why Population Aging Matters: A Global Perspective.* National Institute on Aging, National Institutes of Health March 2007. https://www.nia.nih.gov/research/publication/why-population-aging-matters-global-perspective

Social Science Data Analysis Network. *Trends in Voter Turnout.* University of Michigan SSDAN, 2012. http://www.ssdan.net/sites/default/ files/briefs/vtbrief.pdf

Max Planck Institute for Demographic Research and Vienna Institute of Demography. *The Human Fertility Database.* Joint project of the MPIDR and the VID, based at the MPIDR, Rostock, Germany. http://www. humanfertility.org/cgi-bin/main.php

Tim Kane. *The Importance of Startups in Job Creation and Job Destruction.* Ewing Marion Kauffman Foundation, 2010. http://www. kauffman.org/what-we-do/research/firm-formation-and-growth-series/the-importance-of-startups-in-job-creation-and-job-destruction

Dana P. Goldman, David M Cutler, John W Rowe, Pierre-Carl Michaud, Jeffrey Sullivan, Jay S Olshansky, and Desi Peneva. *Substantial Health and Economic Returns from Delayed Aging May Warrant a New Focus for Medical Research.*" Health Affairs 32 (10) 2013. http://scholar.harvard. edu/cutler/publications/substantial-health-and-economic-returns-delayed-aging-may-warrant-new-focus

Olshansky, S. Jay. *Articulating the Case for the Longevity Dividend.* American Journal of Lifestyle Medicine, 2014. http://ajl.sagepub.com/ content/8/5/336

William W Hung, Joseph S Ross, Kenneth S Boockvar, Albert L Siu. *Recent trends in chronic disease, impairment and disability among older adults in the United States.* BMC Geriatric, 2011. http://www.ncbi.nlm.nih. gov/pmc/articles/PMC3170191/

Papers: Biology

Luigi Fontana, Linda Partridge, Valter D Longo. *Dietary Restriction, Growth Factors and Aging: from yeast to humans.* Science, 2010. http:// www.ncbi.nlm.nih.gov/pmc/articles/PMC3607354/

Nir Barzilai and Ilan Gabriely. *Genetic Studies Reveal the Role of the Endocrine and Metabolic Systems in Aging.* Journal of Clinical

Endocrinology and Metabolism. 2010. http://www.ncbi.nlm.nih.gov/pmc/articles/PMC3050096/

Brian K. Kennedy1, Juniper K. Pennypacker. *Drugs That Modulate Aging: The Promising yet Difficult Path Ahead*. Translational Research, 2014. http://www.ncbi.nlm.nih.gov/pmc/articles/PMC4004650/

Michael F. Holick. *Vitamin D Deficiency*. New England Journal of Medicine 2007. https://www.grc.com/health/pdf/Vitamin_D_Deficiency_Medical_Progress.pdf

Cedric F. Garland, June J. Kim, Sharif B. Mohr, Edward D. Gorham, William B. Grant, Edward L. Giovannucci, Leo Baggerly, Heather Hofflich, Joe W. Ramsdell, Kenneth Zeng, Robert P. Heaney. *Meta-analysis of all-cause mortality according to serum 25-hydroxyvitamin D*. American Journal of Public Health, 2014. http://grassrootshealth.net/media/download/garland2014_ajph_mortality.pdf

Arash Hossein-nezhad, and Michael F. Holick. *Vitamin D for Health: A Global Perspective*. Mayo Clinic Review. http://grassrootshealth.net/media/download/Holick_Mayo_Clinic_Vitamin_D_2013.pdf

Rodrigo A. Cunha, Alexandre de Mendonça. *Therapeutic Opportunities for Caffeine in Alzheimer's Disease and Other Neurodegenerative Diseases*. Journal of Alzheimer's Disease, 2010. http://www.j-alz.com/vol20-supp1

Shinji Saiki, Yukiko Sasazawa, Yoko Imamichi, Sumihiro Kawajiri, Takahiro Fujimaki, Isei Tanida, Hiroki Kobayashi, Fumiaki Sato, Shigeto Sato, Kei-Ichi Ishikawa, Masaya Imoto, Nobutaka Hattori. *Caffeine induces apoptosis by enhancement of autophagy via PI3K/Akt/mTOR/p70S6K inhibition*. Autophagy 2011. https://keio.pure.elsevier.com/en/publications/caffeine-induces-apoptosis-by-enhancement-of-autophagy-via-pi3kak

Zhiwei He, Wei-Ya Ma, Takashi Hashimoto, Ann M. Bode, Chung S. Yang, and Zigang Dong.
Induction of Apoptosis by Caffeine Is Mediated by the p53, Bax, and Caspase 3 Pathways. Journal of Cancer Research, 2003. http://cancerres.aacrjournals.org/content/63/15/4396.short

Francis Bacon. *Novum Organum or True Suggestions for the Interpretation of Nature*. England, 1620. http://www.gutenberg.org/files/45988/45988-h/45988-h.htm

René Vallery-Radot, translated from the French by Mrs. R.L. Devonshire. *The life of Pasteur by René Vallery-Radot*. Doubleday, New York, 1916. https://openlibrary.org/books/OL14020299M/The_life_of_Pasteur

Blanco VM, Chu Z, Vallabhapurapu SD, Sulaiman MK, Kendler A, Rixe O, Warnick RE, Franco RS, Qi X. *Phosphatidylserine-selective targeting and anticancer effects of SapC-DOPS nanovesicles on brain tumors*. Oncotarget 2014. http://www.ncbi.nlm.nih.gov/pubmed/25051370

About the Author

Patrick Cox has lived deep inside the world of technology breakthroughs for the past 30 years. He has written over 200 editorials for *USA Today* and has appeared in the *Wall Street Journal* and on CNN's *Crossfire* television program. In the late 1980s, he edited and published one of the first industry-insider software magazines, writing about topics like open-source and user-supported software long before those ideas were widely understood.

Later, he wrote presentations and speeches for the CEO of Netscape. His consulting work has taken him to Fortune 500 boardrooms and inside the war rooms of national political candidates. His 100% unbiased and independent research is based solely on his investigations in transformational wealth-building companies and close consultation with Nobel Prize-winning economists and scientists.

Patrick is always on the lookout for the next big investment opportunity in biotechnology. You can read his monthly advisory service at www.mauldineconomics.com/tech.

A Long, Healthy Life Is Great—Especially If You Have Money to Spend

Living to a healthy 90 or 100 while enjoying a financially comfortable retirement... that's the dream of most Americans. And with the groundbreaking biotech research described in Patrick Cox's book, both health and wealth can be within your reach.

If you are interested in the anti-aging and life extension research Patrick has spent more than a decade researching, investing in the companies responsible for those potential biotech breakthroughs only makes sense.

As new drugs and therapies move through the FDA-required queue of clinical-trial phases, a successful outcome at any stage can cause a company's stock to rise substantially... sometimes literally overnight.

As a special offer for readers of *The Methuselah Effect*, you can get Patrick Cox's premium alert service, *Transformational Technology Alert*, at a 40% discount. Order online via http://bit.do/patrickcox or simply fill out and send in the coupon below.

As a subscriber, every month you'll receive Patrick and his team's in-depth research on a new therapy or drug with the potential to revolutionize medicine as we know it... along with detailed analysis of the most promising company in that field.

Though biotech is known as a volatile sector, Patrick's strategy of caution and taking profits whenever possible has paid off for his subscribers. To date, all the portfolio stocks that were sold or partially sold have been winners.

As our thank-you for trying *Transformational Technology Alert*, you'll also get three free bonus reports:
- *The Visionary's Guide to Profits: 5 Must-Own Small Biotech Stocks That Could Change the World*
- *Anti-Aging Supplements I Use Now*
- *Shortcuts to Saving Your Life*

Sign Up for Patrick's Free e-Letter Today!

Keep up to date on the latest groundbreaking medical and life extension research—from Zika vaccines to promising new cancer treatments, to spectacular anti-aging therapies—with *Patrick Cox's Tech Digest*. This popular weekly e-letter is brought to you every Thursday, straight to your inbox. Sign up here: http://bit.do/techdigest